DATE DUE

NOV 1 1 2000	
OCT 3 1 2000	
OCT 2 7 2009	
NOV - 9 2009	

GAYLORD   PRINTED IN U.S.A.

Introduction to Long Term Care Nursing:
Principles and Practice

Donna D. Ignatavicius, MS, RNC

Professor
Charles County Community College
School of Nursing
La Plata, Maryland

President
DI Associates
Hughesville, Maryland

 F. A. Davis Company ▪ Philadelphia

F. A. Davis Company
1915 Arch Street
Philadelphia, PA 19103

Printed in the United States of America

Last digit indicates print number: 10 9 8 7 6 5 4 3 2 1

Publisher, Nursing: Robert G. Martone
Nursing Editor: Alan Sorkowitz
Production Editor: Michael Schnee
Cover Designer: Louis J. Forgione

As new scientific information becomes available through basic and clinical research, recommended treatments and drug therapies undergo changes. The author and publisher have done everything possible to make this book accurate, up to date, and in accord with accepted standards at the time of publication. The authors, editors, and publisher are not responsible for errors or omissions or for consequences from application of the book, and make no warranty, expressed or implied, in regard to the contents of the book. Any practice described in this book should be applied by the reader in accordance with professional standards of care used in regard to the unique circumstances that may apply in each situation. The reader is advised always to check product information (package inserts) for changes and new information regarding dose and contraindications before administering any drug. Caution is especially urged when using new or infrequently ordered drugs.

Library of Congress Cataloging-in-Publication Data

Ignatavicius, Donna D.
    Introduction to long-term care nursing : principles and practice /
Donna D. Ignatavicius.
        p.   cm.
    Includes bibliographical references and index.
    ISBN 0-8036-0099-2 (pbk. : alk. paper)
    1. Long-term care of the sick.   2. Geriatric nursing.   I. Title.
    [DNLM: 1. Geriatric Nursing.   2. Long-Term Care—nurses
instruction.   3. Nursing Homes.   WY 152 I241 1998]
    RT120.L64I38   1998
    610.73'65—dc21
    DNLM/DLC
for Library of Congress   97-42724
                                                              CIP

To Norma Shortall, whose mentorship and friendship inspired me to write a book for long term care nurses.

Preface

Nursing students typically care for older adults in many settings, especially nursing homes. New graduate nurses often find their first jobs in nursing homes. Although there are a number of gerontological nursing books available for students and practicing nurses, none seems to focus solely on care of residents in the nursing home setting. Therefore, this book is not a comprehensive text on care of the elderly, but rather an introduction to care in the nursing home for nursing students and nurses new to long term care. Practical, accessible, need-to-know information is found in every chapter.

The major title of the book is *Introduction to Long Term Care Nursing* because the nursing home industry refers to itself as long term care. Although other health care settings may provide long term care, they are not discussed in this text. With the move toward managed care in the United States, some residents are admitted for short term stays and are then discharged to their homes or other settings. Not all residents in nursing homes today require long term care.

Contents of the Book

This book is divided into two major parts. The first part focuses on clinical practice; the second part focuses on issues such as management and quality improvement.

Chapters 1 and 2 introduce the reader to general information about demographics and health care of the elderly, followed by a discussion regarding the characteristics of nursing homes. Chapters 3 through 6 center on the biopsychosocial assessment of the elderly, common health problems seen in nursing home residents, medication use in the elderly, and selected acute illnesses and typical health emergencies.

Chapter 7 describes documentation requirements for nursing home residents. In Chapter 8, health protection and health promotion activities are discussed. The growth of subacute care is addressed in a separate chapter, Chapter 9.

Chapters 10 through 14 cover the structure of the nursing home, the organization and function of the nursing department, the role of the charge nurse in the nursing home, and the survey and quality improvement processes. The last chapter, Chapter 15, highlights the common legal and ethical issues encountered in long term care.

The appendixes provide additional information for the reader, including sample forms, a table on laboratory findings in the elderly, and a description of common complementary therapies that can be used in long term care.

Teaching/Learning Aids

Each chapter has a topical outline and objectives at the beginning, and concludes with a highlighted summary of key points. In addition, the accompanying instructor's guide provides multiple teaching/learning activities.

Instructor's Guide

Faculty will find the *Instructor's Guide* for this book extremely useful. The author, Elaine Bishop Kennedy, believes that critical thinking activities, group work, and cooperative learning are essential teaching/ learning strategies. To that end, she has provided an outline, content description with suggestions for using content for short and longer courses, a list of Internet resources, and multiple critical thinking exercises. Some of the exercises are appropriate as individual written assignments, while others are ideal for group work.

A test bank links each item to a chapter objective. Each item also identifies the correct answer, rationale for the answer, nursing process step (if appropriate), human need category, and cognitive level.

Acknowledgments

To produce a book that meets the needs of nursing students and practicing nurses requires the help and support of a lot of caring people. I especially want to thank the reviewers who provided excellent feedback and ideas for each chapter:

Carolyn Baxter, RN, NHA, CNDLTC
Nursing Home Administrator
Complete Care Services
Horsham, Pennsylvania

Janice Cameron, AAS, BS, MS
Chief Executive Officer
Geriatric Health Care Consultants
Drexel Hill, Pennsylvania

Linda Chamberlain, MS, BSN, RN, CNA, NHA
Director of Special Projects
Wilmac Corporation
Lancaster, Pennsylvania

Rick Cooper, RN, MSN
Assistant Professor
Allegany College of Maryland
Cumberland, Maryland

Grace A. Cumberbatch, RN, MA in Nursing
Associate Professor of Nursing
LaGuardia Community College
Brooklyn, New York

Susan Hauser Jeffers, RN, MS
Instructor
Mansfield General Hospital School of Nursing
Mansfield, Ohio

Gail Ann Kelly, MA, RN
Instructor of Nursing
Nassau Community College
Garden City, New York

Elaine Bishop Kennedy, EdD, RN
Associate Professor, Nursing
Wor-Wic Community College
Cambridge, Maryland

Ferne C. N. Kyba, RN, PhD
Assistant Professor
University of Texas at Arlington
Arlington, Texas

Evelyn Massey-Porter, RN, BSN
Chair, Vocational Nursing
City College of San Francisco
San Francisco, California

Sue Matthews, RN, BSEd
Instructor
South Plains College—Lubbock
Lubbock, Texas

Martina Obenski, RN, MSN
Assistant Professor of Nursing
Cedar Crest College
Allentown, Pennsylvania

Ellen Smet, RN, MSN
formerly Nursing Instructor
Asheville-Buncombe Technical Community College
Asheville, North Carolina

Josephine Stewart, BSN, CRNI
Director of Nursing Education
Infusion Management Systems
Missouri City, Texas

Kendra M. Strenth, RNC, MSN
Coordinator
Bishop State Community College—Southwest Campus
Mobile, Alabama

The staff at F. A. Davis have been great to work with. Their patience, support, and professionalism made my job easier. I owe a special note of thanks to Alan Sorkowitz, Nursing Editor; Bob Martone, Nursing Publisher; Robert Butler, Production Manager; Michael Schnee, Production Editor; and Louis Forgione, Cover Designer.

My husband and daughter, Charles and Stephanie, have been my special support system. Without them, I could not write books or experience the other growth opportunities I have had in my career. I also thank the educators and practitioners around the country who encouraged me and have eagerly awaited the publication of this book.

Contents

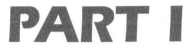

PART I

PATIENT CARE MANAGEMENT IN LONG TERM CARE

1 Health Care of the Elderly: An Overview

OUTLINE

Demographics of Aging
Health Status of the Elderly
Health Care Settings for Elders

OBJECTIVES

- Identify subgroups of the elderly
- Describe the health status of the elderly population
- Identify a variety of settings where elders seek health care

The number of people over 65 years of age in the United States is growing rapidly, currently accounting for more than 13 percent of the population. Many factors contribute to this growth, including the development of technology and potent medications that have increased life expectancy. In less than 15 years, when the "baby boomer" generation becomes elderly, this percentage is expected to double or triple. Worldwide, in 1991 there were nearly half a billion people over 60 years of age (Ebersole & Hess, 1994).

Unfortunately, health care professionals in the past were not educated regarding how to look after the elderly when they needed care. As a result, many myths about the elderly as a group had an adverse influence on the way that health care has been delivered to these individuals. For example, some nurses still believe that the elderly are confused, incontinent, immobile, and dependent in self-care. These beliefs stem from the fact that nurses usually care for people who are ill rather than provide wellness care.

Actually, 80 percent to 85 percent of people over 65 are in relatively stable health, even though they may have one or more chronic diseases. Only 5 percent are living in nursing homes. However, as many as 30 percent to 40 percent may spend some time in a nursing home for short term care. The elderly are typically not confused and are able to care for themselves. However, when some elders become ill and are removed from their comfortable, familiar environment, they experience a number of physical and emotional changes. These are discussed in later chapters of this book.

Demographics of Aging

For many years, the beginning of elderhood was tagged at 65 years of age. In more recent years, researchers have suggested that "late adulthood" begins at 60, or perhaps 55. For the purpose of this clinically oriented book, the elderly will refer to people 65 years of age and older.

SUBGROUPS OF THE ELDERLY

As people age, they become even more individualized than in earlier years. Although both can be considered as elders, a 70-year-old is very different from a 90-year-old. Some 70-year-old elders look like 90-year-olds; conversely, some 90-year-olds look like 70-year-olds. Recognizing this variability, several attempts to divide the elderly into subgroups have been made. One of the most popular classifications is:

- 65 to 74 years old = young old
- 74 to 84 years old = middle old
- 85 to 99 years old = old old
- 100 and above = elite old (centenarians)

Of the above groups, the fastest growing is the old old, followed by the elite old. Many elders over 85 years of age are frail and have multiple health problems (Fig. 1–1). Consequently, this group is most likely to be admitted to a nursing home.

TRANSCULTURAL CONSIDERATIONS

One of the areas regarding elder care that needs to be more directly addressed is the culturally diverse society that exists in the United States. Although the current elderly population is not as diverse as it will be in

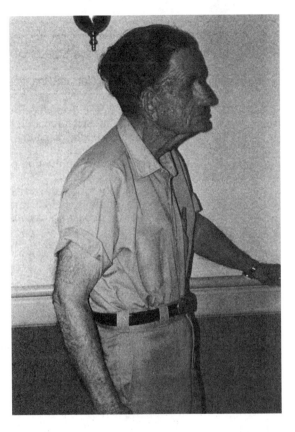

Figure 1–1. *An advanced elderly person in a nursing home. (From* Medical-Surgical Nursing: A Nursing Process Approach, *2nd ed. (p. 58), by D.D. Ignatavicius, M.L. Workman, & M.A. Mishler, 1995, Philadelphia: W.B. Saunders. Reprinted with permission.)*

20 years, cultural differences need to be considered when caring for the elderly.

In general, the life expectancy of African Americans, Native Americans, Mexican Americans, and others of Hispanic descent is less than the life expectancy of Caucasians (Giger & Davidhizar, 1995). Nursing home admission of non-Caucasian groups is also lower than that of Caucasians. In large part, the low admission rate is because the strong family units in these groups feel responsible for the care of their elderly and tend to keep them at home until death.

In addition to ethnic and/or racial variations among the elderly, educational, gender, religious, and socioeconomic differences play a role in their health care. For example, the elderly woman of today may not have a high school education and may continue to rely on her husband for financial support. If she is widowed, she may live on Social Security benefits. Many elderly people have a strong religious and spiritual faith that provides comfort for them in wellness and illness. Chapter 3 discusses spirituality of the elderly in more detail.

Health Status of the Elderly

In 1961, the first White House Conference on Aging directed increased attention to a variety of needs of the growing numbers of elderly in the United States. As a result of this landmark conference, the Older Americans Act was passed by Congress in 1965. This piece of legislation provided for many community services, including food (Meals on Wheels), transportation, and housing. In 1973, the law was amended to create the federal, state, and local Offices for the Aging to coordinate these services.

Providing these community services to anyone over 60 years of age, regardless of financial ability, improved the health status of the elderly, who could then visit the physician for detection or follow-up of health problems. Improved nutrition helped prevent illness and promote healing. These services continue to be available to the elderly.

The health status of an older adult today depends on a number of factors, including socioeconomic status, common health practices, and the incidence of chronic disease. For the person who is retired and living on a fixed income, usually Social Security, health care falls well behind food and housing as a priority. In general, the poorer the individual, the poorer the health status is likely to be. African Americans, Native Americans, and people of Hispanic descent are more likely to have a lower socioeconomic status and therefore a poorer health state than Caucasians (Giger & Davidhizar, 1995).

Health practices vary among the elderly. Again, the economic factor plays a role, in that a person who cannot afford health care is not likely to be engaging in formal health promotion practices like annual physical examinations.

Many elderly do not trust the health care system. Some people still remember when hospitals were a place where very sick people went for treatment and most died, especially before the era of antibiotics. Others fear that they will be placed in a nursing home. To most older adults, nursing home admission represents the "end of the line," a place where they will lose everything, give up, and die.

In view of these fears and anxieties, it is no wonder that when an elder becomes ill, he or she may turn to a spouse or friend for medical advice and perhaps share medication or another treatment modality. Or the individual may seek the advice of a pharmacist at a local drug store for over-the-counter medication for self-treatment.

Those elderly who do trust the health care system and faithfully work with their physician or nurse practitioner generally view these professionals as godlike. Whatever the physician tells them, they believe, and they are, therefore, unlikely to get a second opinion regarding their health state unless they are required to do so by third-party payers (insurance companies). This overwhelming trust of the physician can become a barrier for the nurse who may be teaching elders how to better take care of themselves.

Chronic diseases are much more common in the elderly than in the younger adult. The older the individual, the more predisposed he or she is to diseases like cardiovascular disease, dementias, arthritis, and diabetes mellitus. When these diseases are not controlled, acute episodes or emergencies occur, often with the result that an individual requires hospitalization.

Health Care Settings for Elders

HOSPITALS

The elderly receive health care in a number of settings. In the acute care setting (hospital), between 60 percent and 70 percent of all persons admitted are over 65 years old. Medical-surgical nursing has become acute gerontological nursing. As hospitals continue to downsize and redesign their institutions, their patients are being discharged "sicker and quicker."

The implications of these changes for nursing are fairly obvious. First, nurses must become more educated about how to care for hospitalized elderly. Second, nurses need to begin continuing care teaching and planning at the time of hospital admission. This process is facilitated in settings where case management and clinical pathways are used.

In a case managed environment, a case manager (usually a nurse) follows the patient from before hospital admission, if possible, through discharge, using a clinical pathway as a tool. Other clinical settings, such as home care and nursing homes, are just beginning to use pathways. Chapter 7 discusses clinical pathways and illustrates an example.

In some hospitals, the case manager continues to follow the patient into the nursing home, rehabilitation, or home care setting. Nurses must also know the community services available for the elderly and how they can be accessed. Most hospitals have or are beginning to plan case management systems to improve quality care in a cost-effective manner.

AMBULATORY CARE SETTINGS

Just as the elderly are the primary consumers of health care in hospitals, they are also the primary consumers in many ambulatory settings, such as clinics, same-day surgicenters, and physicians' offices. They are less likely to be part of a health maintenance organization (HMO) because these settings contract with employers and their work force. However, traditional Medicare is converting to managed care Medicare over the next several years.

Like nurses, physicians who have been in practice for a number of years have generally not been educated in the special care associated with the elderly. More physicians than ever before are becoming board-certified geriatricians.

HOME CARE

Many elders are being cared for in their homes or the homes of their family members by caregivers. Most of these caregivers are members of the family and significant others. Some older adults may need to employ an aide or nurse to provide daily care. In other cases, home care nurses and aides employed by a home care agency may make periodic visits to monitor the health status of the elderly person and perform selected treatments or teaching. For elders who are not as physically impaired, adult day care centers offer an opportunity for socialization and respite for the family or other caregiver.

NURSING HOMES

Only a small percentage of elderly people in the United States are in nursing homes. However, an increase in the need for nursing home care is expected as the population ages. The next chapter describes the characteristics of a nursing home in detail.

CHAPTER HIGHLIGHTS

In this book, the elderly refers to persons over 65 years of age.

There are several subgroups of the aged population; the fastest growing group is that over 85 years old.

When compared with Caucasians, the life expectancy rate, nursing home admission rate, and income of African Americans, Native Americans, and people of Hispanic descent are lower.

The Older Americans Act provides transportation, food, and housing for people over 60 years old who need these services.

Chronic disease is most prevalent in people over 65 years old.

Many elderly individuals do not trust the health care system or fear being admitted to a hospital or nursing home.

Elder care occurs in a variety of health care settings, including the hospital, ambulatory care settings, home, and nursing home.

REFERENCES AND READINGS

Anderson, M.A., & Braun, J.V. (1995). *Caring for the elderly client.* Philadelphia: F.A. Davis.
Burke, M.M., & Walsh, M.B. (1997). *Gerontologic nursing.* St. Louis: Mosby.
Ebersole, P., & Hess, P (1994). *Toward healthy aging.* St. Louis: Mosby.
Giger, J.N., & Davidhizar, R.E. (1995). *Transcultural nursing: Assessment and intervention.* St. Louis: C.V. Mosby.
Hines-Martin, V.P. (1992). A research review: Family caregivers of chronically-ill African-American elderly. *Journal of Gerontological Nursing, 18*(2), 25–29.
MacPhail, J. (1993). Intergenerational caring in professional and family life. *Geriatric Nursing, 14*, 104–107.
Ringsven, M.K., & Bond, D. (1997). *Gerontology and leadership skills for nurses.* Albany, NY: Delmar.

DISCUSSION QUESTIONS TO PROMOTE CRITICAL THINKING

1. Based on the increasing elderly population, what would you predict for the future of nursing homes and long term care nursing?
2. What would you predict for the future of community-based nursing?
3. How might the role of nursing change in the twenty-first century as the elderly population increases?

2

Characteristics of Nursing Homes

OBJECTIVES

- Briefly discuss the growth of the nursing home industry
- Differentiate the major types of nursing homes
- Describe the typical nursing home resident
- Define relocation syndrome and its cause
- Identify the major sources of reimbursement for nursing home care

Nursing homes in the United States serve individuals with chronic illnesses and physical impairments. People admitted to a nursing home are residents of that home. As people live longer with more complex health problems, the nursing home industry continues to grow. There are currently more than 1.5 million occupied nursing home beds, which is three times the number of hospital beds, and this number is expected to increase to more than 2 million by the year 2000.

About 80 percent of nursing homes are proprietary, meaning that they are businesses that aim to make a profit. They may be privately owned by small companies or individuals, or corporately owned by large chains, such as Beverly Enterprises. The remaining homes are nonprofit or not-for-profit and government-owned. Chapter 10 discusses ownership in more detail.

History of Nursing Homes

In the 1930s, legislation for the creation of Social Security, housing programs, and welfare provided new sources of income for the elderly. Despite their intent, these programs were not successful in encouraging families to care for their elders at home. Instead, many privately owned, family-run boarding homes were started to provide room, board, and personal care for the elderly. When these homes added nurses to their staff, the homes were called nursing homes, a term that continues to be used commonly today.

Nursing homes began accepting people with more complex chronic problems, and reimbursement for elder care began in the mid-1960s with the passage of Title XVIII (Medicare) and Title XXIX (Medicaid). Under these conditions, the nursing home industry experienced a rapid and unchecked growth spurt that gave rise to abuses. As a result, in the 1970s, a number of criminal charges were filed against nursing home owners for finance and reimbursement fraud, vendor kickbacks, and violations of individuals' rights. These scandals prompted the states to enact laws requiring licensure of all nursing homes, as well as inspections to ensure that these crimes no longer occurred.

Since that time, the media have continued to present a negative image of nursing homes. Large groups of elderly citizens, especially the American Association of Retired Persons (AARP), have lobbied Congress to pass stiffer laws to regulate the care that elderly people receive in nursing homes. In 1987, the Omnibus Budget Reconciliation Act (OBRA) mandated that residents' rights, quality of care, and quality of life be more strictly addressed. Nursing homes had to become more "homelike." New regulations stemming from this piece of federal legislation were enacted on October 1, 1990, and are discussed later in this chapter.

Nature of Nursing Homes and Their Residents

The term "nursing home" is used to describe a number of types of facilities that provide protection and care for the elderly. Long term care (LTC) has become synonymous with nursing home care. Each state determines what types of homes it will license, based on predetermined requirements. Several types are commonly seen in the United States (Table 2–1).

TYPES OF NURSING HOMES

Residential Care Homes

Previously called rest homes, residential facilities usually include domiciliary homes, personal care homes, assisted living facilities, and group homes. They are small and much like the earlier boarding homes operating prior to the creation of Medicare and Medicaid in the mid-1960s. The typical resident of a residential home is able to perform most or all self-care. As residents become more dependent, they are transferred to a traditional nursing home that has 24-hour professional nursing care.

Rest homes have few professional health services and may or may not require licensure, depending upon the state. Most residents either pay out-of-pocket or have their care subsidized by Medicaid or local funding.

Nursing Facilities

Licensed nursing homes may also be certified to designate what level of care they provide and how they may be reimbursed for that care. Nursing homes certified for providing intermediate level care were formerly called intermediate care facilities (ICFs). The newer term is nursing facility (NF).

Table 2–1. **Types of Long Term Care Facilities: Resident Profile**

Type of LTC Facility or Unit	Type of Residents
Residential care	Residents are able to provide most of their own care; personal care may be provided
Nursing facility (NF)	Intermediate care provided; most residents need help with activities of daily living (ADLs)
Skilled nursing facility (SNF)	Skilled care provided by licensed health care professionals
Subacute care	Residents require complex care but are medically stable
Retirement community	Care ranges from independent living to total dependence, depending on need
Specialty unit	Level of care varies; care centered around diagnosis

NFs are usually eligible to receive Medicaid funding, a state reimbursement program, for care of residents who are dependent in a number of activities of daily living (ADLs), although the rules vary somewhat by state. Examples of ADLs include dressing, bathing, and feeding.

Depending upon the state, residents may be classified as light care, moderate care, heavy care, or heavy special care. Light care residents require less assistance with ADLs than residents in the other classifications. Reimbursement for resident care is based on the level or amount of nursing care required.

Some states, such as Texas and Nebraska, have a large number of ICFs, while others, such as California, have very few. Approximately one-third of all nursing home beds are certified as intermediate care (Matteson, McConnell, & Linton, 1997).

Skilled Nursing Facilities

Nursing homes that are certified for Medicare funding, a federal reimbursement program, are called skilled nursing facilities (SNFs, pronounced "snifs"). SNFs provide care that requires the attention of health care professionals, such as nurses, physical therapists, or occupational therapists. While intermediate care focuses on ability to perform ADLs, skilled care focuses on those treatments or therapies that are not usually performed by an unlicensed staff member. Examples might include rehabilitation for a fractured hip, tube feedings, and ostomy care. Medicare pays for only a small portion of nursing home resident care—about 2 percent.

Some states have a unique licensing and certification procedure that combines intermediate and skilled care. For example, in Maryland, nursing home beds may be designated as comprehensive, meaning that a resident requiring intermediate or skilled care can be admitted to any bed in the facility.

Retirement Communities

Some nursing homes are a part of a larger complex known as a retirement community or center. These centers may be either life care retirement communities (LCRCs) or continuing care retirement communities (CCRCs). Both types tend to have independent living housing, such as apartments and/or cottages, as well as a nursing home that is available if the resident needs temporary or permanent care. The nursing home beds may be intermediate, skilled, or a combination. Some centers also have an assisted living (or domiciliary) area for residents who need 24-hour supervision but not necessarily 24-hour nursing care.

In the life care centers, the resident usually pays a large admission fee that covers living expenses and nursing home care for as long as needed. In continuing care centers, the resident typically pays a smaller admission fee but pays monthly for the level of care required.

Extended Care Facilities

The concept of extended care facilities (ECFs) was not intended to be the same as that of the nursing home. The idea of ECFs was developed for hospitals who wanted a longer term unit for patients being discharged from the acute area. This type of facility is not widely used, although the term ECF is sometimes still used.

Specialty Care

Over the past 10 years, many types of specialty units have been developed as part of the nursing home or as freestanding units. In these units, all residents have the same or similar medical diagnoses. Some of the most common are dementia or geropsychiatric units, head injury units, and ventilator units.

A dementia unit admits residents who have a diagnosis of dementia, usually Alzheimer's disease. The advantage of this type of unit is that care can be specifically tailored to meet the special needs of these residents. For instance, activities for demented residents need to be structured differently from those for residents who are not demented. The staff ratio may need to be higher than in the traditional nursing home unit because, depending on the stage of the disease, more intense supervision may be needed.

As described in Chapter 4 in the section on dementia, residents with dementia need environmental structuring. The unit must be safe, comfortable, and not overstimulating. One of the problems with having a dementia unit is establishing admission and discharge criteria. Some units try to admit residents with early to middle stages of dementia. But many families want to keep their loved ones at home until the emotional behavior or physical condition becomes too difficult to be handled by a caregiver in the home.

Other units admit individuals in any stage of dementia. Families of residents with early to middle stage dementia may not want their loved one in the same unit as those residents with late stage disease. In spite of these and other dilemmas, dementia units are fairly popular and continue to develop as the number of elderly with dementia increases.

The residents in head injury and "vent" units tend to be young and middle-aged adults rather than the elderly. Many states reimburse the nursing home at a higher rate for these residents, who are sicker or require more complex care.

Another special purpose of a nursing home is respite care. The most common site for institutional respite care is the nursing home (Stanley & Beare, 1995). Although not generally reimbursed by third-party payers, such as Medicare or Medicaid, respite care provides an opportunity for a family to admit a loved one to a nursing home on a temporary basis while they "take a break" from their caregiving duties for that person at home. Some nursing homes have designated respite care beds to use for that purpose.

Subacute Care

Subacute care is the newest concept in care for people who require complex health care but who are medically stable enough to be discharged from the hospital. These patients are usually too ill to be cared for in a home setting or do not have family support for caregiving at home. Chapter 9 describes subacute care in more detail.

NATURE OF NURSING HOME RESIDENTS

The Elderly Resident

In most nursing homes, the typical nursing home resident is a widowed, Caucasian female over 80 years old. There is a preponderance of women because women outlive men (Fig. 2–1). Caucasian elders usually have less family support than most other ethnic and/or racial groups and therefore need nursing home placement. African American and Asian American families, for example, have greater reverence for their elders than

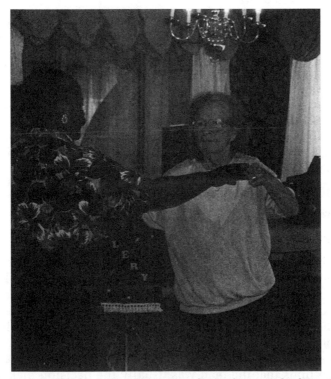

Figure 2–1. An active elderly woman in a nursing home. (From Medical-Surgical Nursing: A Nursing Process Approach, *2nd ed. (p. 47), by D.D. Ignatavicius, M.L. Workman, & M.A. Mishler, 1995, Philadelphia: W.B. Saunders. Reprinted with permission.)*

Caucasians and often care for the elders in the home until death (Giger & Davidhizar, 1995).

Although the elderly predominate in the nursing home population, several recent findings are of interest. First, two groups of elderly residents seem to be emerging—the short-term and long-term groups. The short-term resident typically is under 75 years of age and stays in the facility for 2 to 6 weeks for rehabilitation of acute illnesses, such as strokes, total hip and knee replacements, and fractures. The traditional long-term resident is older, has numerous chronic diseases, and has more cognitive and functional impairments. Long-term residents outnumber short-term residents 9 to 1, but this ratio is changing as a result of managed care.

Long-term residents have an average stay of about 2½ years and experience heart disease, dementia (two-thirds of all residents), arthritis, and diabetes mellitus. Most of this group die in the nursing home or in the hospital with an acute illness. Between 85 percent and 90 percent of nursing home residents have some type of sensory impairment, such as vision and hearing deficits (Matteson, McConnell, & Linton, 1997).

The Younger Resident

Another new trend is the increase in admissions of younger residents with chronic diseases to nursing homes. As health care and technology have improved, people who formerly died from diseases early in life are now living longer. Some common examples are diseases such as multiple sclerosis, Huntington's disease, and muscular dystrophy. Individuals with these illnesses often require total care and are unable to stay in the home due to limited resources for caregiving. The husband, wife, or significant other often cannot provide total care because he or she must work to maintain an income. Hiring appropriate around-the-clock caregivers is difficult in many cases and very costly.

THE TRANSITION TO NURSING HOME CARE

Family Dynamics

Making the decision regarding nursing home admission is usually very difficult for the family. Although families today are caring for loved ones with more complex health problems than ever before, the family may have no choice but to turn to nursing home care as an alternative. Nursing home admission may be the result of lack of family support, inadequate finances, or deteriorating health.

When examining the history of traditional family dynamics of today's elderly, one finds that the man was usually the decision maker until he retired. Then the woman took charge and began to make more of the decisions. Many of today's elderly are being cared for by their elderly daughters or daughters-in-law. It is not unusual to see a 90-year-old woman living with her 70-year-old daughter and her son-in-law, if he is living.

Another common picture is that of the middle-aged woman who is caring for elderly parents or in-laws while completing the rearing of her children. These middle-aged adults are part of a growing "sandwich generation."

Relocation Syndrome

Whether an elderly person or couple sell a house to move into a retirement community or are admitted to a nursing home, relocation is typically very difficult. The more sudden or unexpected the change, the harder it is for an elderly person to adjust. Therefore, slow and gradual planning for relocation, if possible, helps to make the transition smoother.

Most of the literature on relocation focuses on admission to a nursing home, the most drastic environmental change for an older person. When the elderly are removed from their comfortable, familiar environment into a new location, such as a nursing home, behavioral or emotional problems are common. Examples of behaviors that the nurse may observe are memory deficits, acute confusion (or increased confusion), increased anxiety, psychotic syndromes (such as hallucinations), and decreased trust or paranoia. These behaviors contribute to negative health outcomes such as falls and decreased mobility.

In some cases, relocation has been associated with mortality. More subtle changes that have been reported include isolation, passive behavior, and decreased interpersonal communication (Matteson, McConnell, & Linton, 1997).

The highest risk factors that contribute to the negative effects of relocation include lack of preparation before the move; radical environmental change; and being older, male, dependent with respect to ADLs, and cognitively impaired. Studies to validate these factors are inconsistent, but anecdotal accounts seem to strongly associate them with poorer relocation outcomes.

Finance and Reimbursement Issues in Nursing Homes

Although Medicare pays most of the hospital care costs for people over 65, it pays only a small percentage of nursing home care. Most nursing home care is paid for "out-of-pocket" by the resident or family, and residents whose care is paid for in this way are sometimes referred to as private pay residents.

MEDICAL ASSISTANCE REIMBURSEMENT

When personal funds are depleted, the resident may be eligible for Medicaid (medical assistance), a last resort measure for reimbursement. This program does not pay 100 percent of nursing home costs. The resident's monthly Social Security check as well as any other pensions or income are used to help pay the monthly nursing home bill.

The average nursing home bill in the United States is approximately $3000 per month, but the charge for care depends on the type of facility and geographic area. The facility does not get reimbursed from Medicaid at its private pay rate. For instance, a daily room and board cost may be $110, but Medicaid may only pay $85 a day. This difference explains why most nursing homes want a mix of private pay and Medicaid residents. To add to the frustration of a lower reimbursement rate, facilities may have to wait as long as 2 years to receive payment. In other words, resident care delivered in June 1995 may not be reimbursed until some time in 1997. Again, each state varies on rates, how they are paid, and who can qualify for the program.

MEDICARE REIMBURSEMENT

Although Medicare is a federal program for the elderly and the disabled of any age, some variations exist. Several intermediaries, or large insurance companies, have been given the responsibility of making Medicare payments to nursing homes certified to accept Medicare residents. Examples of intermediaries are Mutual of Omaha and Blue Cross/Blue Shield. These companies interpret the rules about reimbursement and make the decision as to whether or not the care should be paid for using Medicare funds.

Currently, as a general requirement, a resident may be eligible for Medicare reimbursement in a nursing home if the resident first has a 3-day qualifying stay in a hospital and requires ongoing skilled care. As Medicare becomes managed care, this requirement may not be necessary. The resident must be certified as Medicare eligible by the facility's utilization committee upon admission, 14 days after admission, and 30 days after admission. If the resident continues to be in need of skilled care after this time, the committee can recertify the resident every 30 days for a maximum of 100 days of care.

State and Federal Regulations Governing Nursing Home Care

For a number of years, states were the primary regulators of the quality of care required in nursing homes. Some states were more stringent than others. As a result, some homes provided poor quality of care, a situation that captured media attention and led to a public outcry for better control. As of October 1, 1990, the landmark Omnibus Budget Reconciliation Act (OBRA) of 1987 was enacted. This law and its associated regulations written by the Health Care Financing Administration (HCFA) addressed quality of care issues that had been ignored in some states for both intermediate and skilled facilities.

Although tougher federal legislation is now in place, each state continues to have its own regulations, which may be stricter than the federal laws. The nursing home is obligated to follow both federal and state regulations, as well as local rules regarding health care facilities. Nursing homes that do not comply with OBRA and state regulations may be fined or possibly lose their licensure and certification status. Every 12 to 18 months, a team of state surveyors arrives unannounced at each nursing home for a multi-day inspection.

The survey process is supposed to focus on resident outcomes, but often also includes a paperwork review and building inspection. In the surveyors' judgment, if a regulation is not being met "consistently" or if there is a "significant" deviation from the regulation, the facility receives a written deficiency report for each regulation with which it is not in compliance. In other words, the nursing home "gets cited" for operations the surveyors feel are not being conducted in accord with federal and state regulations. Federal surveyors sometimes inspect the performance of the state surveyors such that a facility may have two survey teams present at one time or following one another.

Although there are a number of checks and balances in the survey system, including extensive surveyor training, some excellent facilities receive deficiency reports, while poor facilities may be given many chances to improve care enough to satisfy the surveyors. A recent study by the American College of Health Care Administrators found that surveyors incorrectly cited 33 percent of the most serious deficiencies (Erickson, 1995).

For any deficiency listed, the nursing home administrator responds with a proposed plan of correction that must be returned to the state. This plan must be implemented within the designated time frame. All deficiencies with their plan of correction must be posted in a public place in the nursing home. Chapter 13 describes the survey process in detail.

Accreditation of Nursing Homes

Although the licensing process is mandatory for the nursing home to initiate and remain in operation, some homes choose to also apply for voluntary accreditation by the Joint Commission on Accreditation of Healthcare

Organizations (JCAHO). This group was originally created for accreditation of hospitals but has expanded to accredit nursing homes, home health agencies, and others. Only a small percentage of nursing homes are JCAHO accredited. The facility must pay a fee for the JCAHO inspection to determine if the home is following JCAHO standards. The advantage of accreditation for the facility is the ability to be eligible for research grants and training for medical students and residents. Some nursing homes feel that the additional accreditation adds credibility to the facility's image and makes it more marketable to the health care consumer.

The Nursing Home as an Organization

Nursing homes are either freestanding, part of a retirement community, or, less often, a unit in a hospital. They range in size from fewer than 25 to more than 600 beds, although most have between 100 and 200 beds. Nursing homes may be privately owned by a single person or group, or may be part of a small or large corporation, or chain of nursing homes. These variables greatly affect the organization of a facility and its resources.

Each nursing home has a nursing home administrator (NHA) who is responsible for the financial and day-to-day operation of the facility. The NHA reports to the owner, board of directors, or corporate officer.

Within the nursing home are many departments that either provide direct care to residents or provide support services. The largest department is the nursing department, which provides 24-hour resident care. Chapter 10 discusses the role of each department in detail.

Implications for Long Term Care Nursing

Long term care nurses are employed in many different types and sizes of nursing homes. Before deciding on what nursing home to work in, a nurse needs answers to several questions:

- Does the mission and philosophy of the facility focus on high quality resident care in a homelike environment?
- What is the ownership of the nursing home?
- What have been the results of the past few surveys?
- Does the facility have a good reputation in the community for providing high quality care?
- What is the case mix of the residents (both financially and medically)?

The answers to all of these questions affect nursing practice. For example, if a home is owned by a large corporation, corporate human resources for consultation are readily available. However, creating change may be more difficult in a large organization.

Another concern is the issue of case mix. If the facility has a large private pay resident population, more financial resources may be available for support services, equipment, supplies, and so forth. If, on the other hand, the facility is largely Medicaid, fewer resources may be on hand for necessary items.

CHAPTER HIGHLIGHTS

Medicare and Medicaid were enacted in the mid-1960s and promoted a growth spurt in the nursing home industry.

Intermediate care facilities (ICFs) are usually eligible for Medicaid reimbursement for resident care.

Skilled nursing facilities (SNFs) provide skilled care that is given by health care professionals; SNFs are reimbursed by Medicare for skilled care.

Retirement communities, specialty units, and subacute units are new areas within long term care that are rapidly growing.

The typical nursing home resident is a widowed, Caucasian female over 80 years old.

Younger residents (under 65 years of age) are also admitted to nursing homes for chronic illnesses such as multiple sclerosis.

People are admitted to nursing homes primarily because they have no or minimal family support.

Relocation syndrome is common in the elderly, especially when moving from home into a nursing home.

REFERENCES AND READINGS

Erickson, J. (1995). Assessment, survey, enforcement to dominate 1995. *McKnight's Long-Term Care NEWS, 16*(1), 18.

Giger, J.N., & Davidhizar, R.E. (1995). *Transcultural nursing: Assessment and intervention.* St. Louis: Mosby Year Book.

Matteson, M.A., McConnell, E.S., & Linton, A.D. (1997). *Gerontological nursing: Concepts and practice* (2nd ed.). Philadelphia: W.B. Saunders.

Stanley, M., & Beare, P.G. (1995). *Gerontological nursing.* Philadelphia: F.A. Davis.

DISCUSSION QUESTIONS TO PROMOTE CRITICAL THINKING

1. What interventions would help residents in making a transition from their home environment to the nursing home setting?
2. What special needs could you anticipate for younger nursing home residents and how could these be addressed?
3. If you were designing a dementia unit, what environmental concerns would you consider? (You may want to refer to Chapter 4 for help in answering this question)

Assessment of the Nursing Home Resident

OBJECTIVES

- Describe the major physiologic changes associated with aging
- Identify changes in laboratory test values that are affected by aging
- Discuss psychosocial changes associated with aging
- Describe the process for assessment of a newly admitted resident

Assessment of the resident is the first step of the nursing process and determines how care is planned and carried out. Because the majority of residents in a nursing home are over 65, the nurse needs to know some of the typical physical and psychosocial assessment findings that are seen in elderly individuals. Although physiologic changes are common in older adults, not everyone ages at the same rate, and findings are variable from person to person. The following discussion presents some of the changes that *can* occur in elderly residents as a normal part of the aging process.

Physiologic Changes Associated with Aging

Most of the common physiologic changes associated with aging can be characterized as tissue degeneration or losses in tissue elasticity. These changes often predispose the elderly to acute and chronic illnesses.

CARDIOVASCULAR SYSTEM

As a person ages, the heart muscle loses some of its elastic properties and the heart valves become thick and rigid, causing a decreased stroke volume. Because the resting heart rate is not altered, decreased cardiac output then results. When at rest, the older adult does not experience symptoms, such as shortness of breath, because his or her activity level is usually lower than it was in younger years. However, when the older adult person exercises, the heart rate increases and remains elevated for a longer time than when the individual was younger. Also, during illness or other stress, cardiac reserve is diminished and the elderly person can experience tachycardia, fatigue, or even heart failure.

Electrocardiographic changes result from a less efficient and slower conduction system in the heart. Typical changes include decreased voltage of all waves and prolonged intervals, such as a prolonged PR interval (Eliopoulos, 1990).

The blood vessels also become less elastic (arteriosclerosis). The results of this change include an increase in systolic blood pressure, decreased peripheral circulation, especially to the feet, and orthostatic hypotension. In orthostatic hypotension, a decrease in the systolic pressure of more than 20 mm Hg and/or a decrease in the diastolic pressure of more than 10 mm Hg and occurs when the individual changes from a sitting or lying position to a standing position. The sclerosed (hardened) vessels cannot function to push blood to the brain, and the individual is at risk of dizziness or syncope (blackout episodes). Orthostatic hypotension is a major contributing factor to falls in the elderly.

RESPIRATORY SYSTEM

The alveoli of the lungs are ordinarily elastic, inflating on inspiration and partially deflating on expiration. As one ages, the elastic properties of the alveoli (elastic recoil) diminish, trapping air and mucus. Gas exchange is reduced and the older adult experiences a decreased arterial oxygen level (PaO_2).

The depth of respirations is also affected by decreased respiratory muscle function due to atrophy of skeletal muscle fibers. Abdominal accessory muscles cannot be used to help with breathing because they, too, become weaker. The rib cage and thoracic spine may become more rigid due to calcification of cartilage, further compromising respiratory function. In thin, petite Caucasian women, loss of bone mass from the vertebral spine (osteoporosis) leads to severe kyphosis (stooped posture). This abnormal posturing decreases lung inflation (Fig. 3–1).

Another important change in older adults is the decreased function of the cilia and cough reflex. Cilia are fine, hairlike projections in the nose and upper airway that ordinarily filter debris and dust. Together with the cough and gag reflex, the cilia help prevent potential irritants from entering the lungs. To add to this loss of protection, the decreased flow of body fluids typically seen in the elderly prevents removal of dry mucus. The result of these changes is an increased possibility for infections.

NEUROLOGIC/SENSORY SYSTEM

As a person ages, many neurons are lost and brain weight decreases by as much as 5 percent to 7 percent (Eliopoulos, 1990). Reaction time and balance are impaired; deep tendon reflexes are diminished, especially in the lower extremities; and tactile sensation (touch) is decreased.

Although cognition (intellect, judgment, memory) is not impaired as a result of the normal aging process, the teaching-learning process is somewhat affected. The ability to learn remains the same as in younger years, but the elderly person may take longer to learn new material and need more reinforcement.

Other senses are also affected. For example, the ability to taste bitter, sour, salt, and sweet all diminish. The ability to see close objects is also decreased, a condition called presbyopia. The pupils decrease in size, the lens become less transparent, and night vision and tearing decrease. A grayish-yellow ring, caused by lipids, may form around the iris—a change known as arcus senilis.

Presbycusis is the hearing impairment commonly experienced by the older adult; characteristically, the hearing loss is primarily for high-pitched sounds. In addition, because of a decrease in the availability of body fluids, hardened cerumen is likely to accumulate in the ears, causing a conductive hearing loss if cerumen impaction occurs.

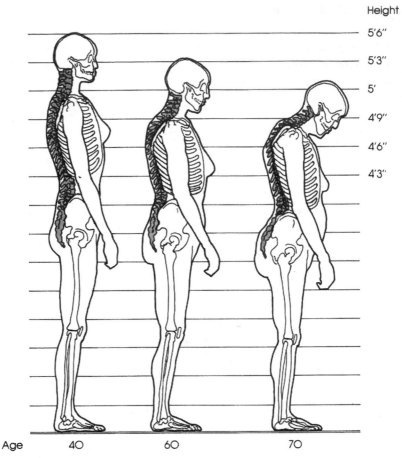

Figure 3–1. *Process of kyphosis in osteoporosis. (From* Medical-Surgical Nursing: A Nursing Process Approach, *2nd ed. (p. 1414), by D.D. Ignatavicius, M.L. Workman, & M.A. Mishler, 1995, Philadelphia: W.B. Saunders. Reprinted with permission.)*

As people age, they tend to sleep less, and total sleep time in the elderly is usually 6 to 7 hours or less per night. In addition, stage IV sleep, in which rapid eye movements (REM) occur, diminishes. REM sleep is an important stage of the sleep cycle for memory, learning, and problem solving, and is the part of the sleep cycle during which dreams occur. Although the significance of having less REM sleep is not completely understood, emotional and behavioral disturbances may result from a decrease in the amount of REM sleep. The elderly person has more frequent awakenings as well.

As people age, the hypothalamus is less responsive to the need for fluid and, consequently, the thirst response diminishes. With decreased total body fluids and a decreased thirst response, elderly individuals can become easily dehydrated.

GASTROINTESTINAL SYSTEM

A number of changes affecting the gastrointestinal (GI) system are seen in the elderly. The teeth are worn, but older adults do not lose teeth from aging. The edentulous (no teeth) elderly of today had no or little preventive dental care in their younger years and have experienced the consequences of poor dental care.

The entire GI tract slows because of diminished elasticity. Secretion of gastric acids decreases, and constipation is common. The production of digestive enzymes also diminishes, including those secreted by the pancreas and small intestines. The liver becomes smaller and reduced in storage and functional capacity.

MUSCULOSKELETAL SYSTEM

Up until age 35, bone tissue is continually breaking down bone (osteoclastic activity) and forming new bone (osteoblastic activity). However, as a person begins middle adulthood, the amount of bone breaking down exceeds the amount of new bone formed. The net result is loss of bone mass. This process is further accelerated in women after menopause and results in the condition known as osteoporosis. After menopause, estrogen, which helps to prevent bone breakdown, declines. Unfortunately, osteoporosis is an irreversible process and is most common in small women of Caucasian origin. African American women generally have more bone stock or reserve and do not commonly experience severe osteoporosis (Ignatavicius, Workman, & Mishler, 1995).

After age 70, osteoporosis leads to multiple fractures, especially compression fractures of the vertebral column, Colles' fracture of the wrist (distal radius), and hip fractures. Men are also susceptible to these problems, but usually after age 80. Until that time, men are protected by testosterone, which actually builds bone.

Synovial joints are also affected by aging. The cartilage that covers the bone ends of each joint begins to degenerate, giving rise to a condition known as degenerative joint disease (DJD) or osteoarthritis. DJD causes pain and decreased mobility, which can lead to a decreased ability to perform self-care.

INTEGUMENTARY SYSTEM

Aging causes many changes in the skin. The epidermal and dermal layers of the skin become thinner, less elastic, and drier. Skin wrinkling and drooping eyelids result from decreased elasticity. Bruising is common because capillaries become fragile. The number of capillaries declines, making the skin more pale (Anderson & Braun, 1995). A decrease in blood supply to the skin also slows the healing process.

Benign "age spots" due to clustering of melanocytes appear on the skin, especially in sun-exposed areas. Although the hair thins and becomes grayer, hair in the nose, eyebrows, and ears becomes thicker. Facial hair also increases in women. Nails are thicker, yellowed, and brittle, with accentuated longitudinal lines.

Loss of subcutaneous tissue and a decline in immune function drop normal body temperature to as low as 96° F. The elderly person is not able to tolerate cold or hot days. When the temperature is hot, the older adult is prone to heat-related illness such as heat exhaustion. When exposed to cold temperatures, the individual may readily experience hypothermia.

RENAL/URINARY SYSTEM

Like the brain, the kidneys lose some of their functional units—the nephrons. Glomerular filtration rate declines, and the ability to concentrate urine may decrease. These changes are probably due to decreased renal blood flow caused by arteriosclerosis of renal arteries.

The urinary bladder capacity becomes smaller, and the detrusor muscle of the bladder weakens. The pelvic floor muscles and urinary sphincter also weaken, resulting in urinary frequency, nocturia (voiding at night), and possibly stress incontinence. Stress incontinence is especially common in elderly obese women who have had multiple children. Dribbling of a small amount of urine occurs when intra-abdominal pressure increases, such as during coughing, sneezing, or straining at stool.

Men also experience incontinence if they have benign prostatic hyperplasia (BPH). BPH causes urethral constriction and urinary retention. The urine may continuously dribble around the enlarged prostate—a condition known as overflow incontinence.

REPRODUCTIVE SYSTEM

As women pass through menopause, estrogen production declines. The results of decreased estrogen on the reproductive system are ovarian atrophy, dry vagina, thinned pubic hair, and decreased breast size. Breasts also sag because skin loses some of its elasticity.

The vagina narrows and loses some of its elasticity as well. Secretions become more alkaline, making the woman more prone to vaginitis. Sexual intercourse can be uncomfortable unless lubrication is applied. Women often have intercourse less frequently as they age because they generally outlive their male partners.

Men also experience changes in their reproductive organs. Although testosterone production does not decrease until 80 years of age or older, the testes decrease in size and firmness. The ability to have an erection and to ejaculate continues, but activities may be slower and less forceful.

Laboratory Test Values Affected by Aging

The normal values for laboratory tests are based upon those ranges common in young adults between 20 and 40 years of age (see Appendix A). "Normal" values for people over 65 have not yet been completely determined. However, param-eters for a few common tests have been established (Table 3–1). This very new information has not been widely disseminated, and it is likely that many health care professionals are not yet aware of these new determinations.

HEMATOLOGIC TESTS

Aging can affect the ability of bone marrow to produce adequate and effectively functioning blood cells. For example, the red blood cell count, hemoglobin, and hematocrit are often lower than that of younger adults. Older men are more likely than older women to have these findings because the production of androgens diminishes with aging.

The immune response in the elderly is also affected. The total white blood cell (WBC) count decreases slightly. The number of lymphocytes, which give rise to antibodies, declines, so that the elderly are predisposed to infections and other immune-related diseases, such as cancer. The function of the cells may also be less effective.

Table 3–1. **Changes in Selected Laboratory Values with Aging**

Laboratory Test	**Change in Values**
Red blood cell count, hemoglobin, and hematocrit	Decreased (especially in women)
White blood cell count	Decreased (especially lymphocytes)
Thyroid hormones (T_3, T_4)	Decreased
Serum iron and vitamin B_{12}	Decreased
Serum glucose	Increased
Blood urea nitrogen (BUN)	Increased
Alkaline phosphatase, creatine kinase (CK), alanine aminotransferase (ALT)	Increased
Serum calcium	Decreased
Creatinine clearance	Decreased

BLOOD CHEMISTRIES

Other substances necessary for red blood cell production, such as iron and vitamin B_{12}, decrease as individuals age. Serum iron may drop to as much as 50 percent to 70 percent of the young adult level. By age 70, the vitamin B_{12} level may decrease by as much as 50 percent (Tietz, 1995).

Decreased endocrine function results in reduced production of several hormones. For example, diminished insulin production leads to a mild elevation of serum glucose. Thyroid hormones, especially triiodothyronine (T_3) and thyroxin (T_4), which are necessary for body metabolism, decline by as much as 25 percent.

As described earlier in this chapter, kidney function also diminishes with aging. The result is that blood urea nitrogen (BUN), a waste product of protein metabolism, can increase to as much as 69 mg/dL (Ignatavicius, Workman, & Mishler, 1995). BUN, however, is not the most reliable indicator of renal function. It can also be elevated as a result of increased protein intake, increased protein catabolism (especially in states of immobility), and dehydration. Serum creatinine, another protein waste product, is the most reliable indicator of renal function and may be slightly elevated in the elderly.

Serum enzymes may also be elevated as a result of aging because many types of tissues undergo degeneration and atrophy. Examples of enzymes with elevated levels include alkaline phosphatase, total creatine kinase (CK), and alanine aminotransferase (ALT), formerly called serum glutamic-pyruvic transaminase (SGPT).

Petite, elderly women at risk for osteoporosis typically have a lowered serum calcium level. The parathyroid glands attempt to compensate for this imbalance by pulling calcium out of the bone, leaving the bones brittle and vulnerable to fracture (Lee, Barrett, & Ignatavicius, 1996).

CREATININE CLEARANCE

Evaluation of creatinine clearance (CrCl), a urine test, reveals a decline in the ability of the kidneys to rid the body of creatinine. CrCl can be measured directly by using a 24-hour urine collection or can be estimated using the following formula (for men):

$$CrCl = \frac{(140 - age) \times body\ weight\ (in\ kg)}{72 \times serum\ creatinine\ (mg/dL)}$$

For women, the result is then multiplied by 0.85.

To illustrate the difference in creatinine clearance between a young adult and older adult, a 20-year-old man weighing 70 kg (154 lb) and having a serum creatinine of 1.0 mg/dL has a CrCl of approximately 117 mL/min.

The CrCl of a 70-year old man with the same weight and serum creatinine drops to 68 mL/min.

Of all of the laboratory changes associated with aging, the creatinine clearance has the most important clinical significance. Most medications are excreted via the kidneys. As the CrCl declines, the kidneys are less able to rid the body of the drug and, consequently, drug toxicities in the elderly are common. An individual must have adequate renal function to take medication that is excreted by the kidneys.

ARTERIAL BLOOD GASES

Because the elderly experience changes in the lungs, especially in the alveoli, diffusion of oxygen into the bloodstream, and of carbon dioxide out of the bloodstream, diminishes. The result is a lowered arterial oxygen level and a slightly increased carbon dioxide level.

Psychosocial Changes Associated with Aging

LOSSES IN LATE ADULTHOOD

Many view late adulthood as a time of losses. Indeed, many elderly do experience one or more losses, although some losses may have occurred in middle adulthood. Some older adults are able to cope well with these losses in a positive way, while others dwell on them and can become clinically depressed.

Many people retire from their career or job at the age of 65. Some individuals adapt to this change in lifestyle and look forward to being able to do things they hadn't had time for while they were working. Others have a difficult adjustment to retirement because they identify themselves by their career or work role. To this group, retirement is viewed as a loss rather than an opportunity.

Another common psychosocial change is loss of a loved one, especially a spouse. For the woman, this loss is particularly difficult because she most likely did not handle the finances or have a separate source of income. Most adult children tend to be supportive during family crises, however, and assist in the adjustment process to the extent possible.

In late adulthood, friends become ill and may either die or be admitted to a nursing home. Loss of or compromised health is another change that may be faced.

For some elderly couples, widows, or widowers, loss of a house occurs if they decide to move into a more protected environment, such as a retirement complex. This relocation can be traumatic and may be viewed as a major loss.

Admission to a nursing home is a particularly difficult adjustment. Chapter 2 discusses relocation syndrome as a result of nursing home admission. The nurse assessing the resident must be aware that this adjustment can alter assessment findings.

NEW ROLES IN LATE ADULTHOOD

Although many elderly people experience multiple losses, becoming older also offers a chance to develop and enjoy new roles. For example, grandparenting and great-grandparenting can be very enjoyable roles (Fig. 3–2). Having leisure time may afford the opportunity to travel, take up a new hobby, or perform community service.

SPIRITUALITY IN LATE ADULTHOOD

Spirituality is not the same as religion, although religion is one way of expressing spirituality. Spiritual needs are broader and include hope, love, faith, and a meaning to life. Some researchers have investigated the importance of religion and religious beliefs during late adulthood. Koenig (1987) studied more than 1000 individuals between 55 and 94 years of age in a Midwest community. His conclusions were:

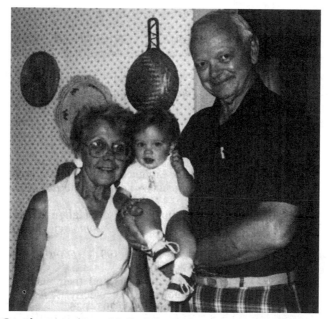

Figure 3–2. Grandparents. (From Medical-Surgical Nursing: A Nursing Process Approach, 2nd ed. (p. 59), by D.D. Ignatavicius, M.L. Workman, & M.A. Mishler, 1995, Philadelphia: W.B. Saunders. Reprinted with permission.)

- A large number of individuals found that religion helped them to cope during stressful life events.
- Religious beliefs and activities were prevalent among older adults.
- A strong relationship exists between well-being and religion, especially for women older than 75 years.

The church is also a social institution, and for many churches, between 40 percent and 60 percent of the congregants are over 65 years of age (Ebersole & Hess, 1994). Parish nursing is becoming a growing field in which churches, sometimes in collaboration with hospitals, are providing health promotion functions for the elderly.

Keeping the role of religion and spirituality in mind, it is apparent that the resident in a nursing home continues to have spiritual needs that must be met. On admission, the nurse needs to ask about religious affiliation, as well as other ways in which spiritual needs can be met, such as having related reading material available.

Assessment of Residents in Young and Middle Adulthood

YOUNG ADULTHOOD

Younger residents have special needs and concerns as they pass through young and middle adulthood. Young adulthood is generally designated as encompassing the years between 18 and 35 years of age. In this stage of development, the sense of self-identity becomes clearer. Entrance into the work world involves selection of a career or occupation, as well as providing an opportunity for socialization.

Interpersonal relationships are more meaningful in young adulthood as compared to adolescence. Fulfillment of sexual needs is also increasingly important.

The major milestone is usually family involvement or expansion. Of course, not all young adults marry or have children.

Transcultural Considerations

There are generally two types of family structures. One is patriarchal (headed by men) and the other is matriarchal (headed by women). About half of all African American families are matriarchal, compared to one-fourth of families of Hispanic origin and one-sixth of Caucasian families (Giger & Davidhizar, 1995).

Impact of Nursing Home Admission on Young Adults

Young adults may be admitted to a nursing home for a number of reasons, including strokes; work-or leisure-related accidents, such as head and spinal cord injuries; degenerative neurologic diseases, such as multiple sclerosis and Huntington's disease; and sickle cell disease. Very little has been written about the effect of nursing home placement on young adults. Certainly young adults may feel isolated in a facility where most other residents are significantly older. Some have families or significant others who need to be part of the assessment and planning process. Others are in the nursing home because there is no family support. An essential part of the assessment is to determine how young adults feel about placement, so that interventions can be planned that meet their specific needs. These interventions include aggressive discharge planning to locate another level of care or setting where these individuals can be with more of their peers.

MIDDLE ADULTHOOD

The middle years between young and later adulthood have often been referred to as the best years of adult life—the "prime of life" (Fig. 3–3). Middlescence (middle age) is the time, though, when people realize that they are at the midpoint in their lives. Some individuals respond negatively to this age and experience a "mid-life crisis," unable to cope with the reality that they are getting older. Many of the physiologic changes associated with aging, and discussed earlier, begin during middle adulthood.

Nursing home admission of the middle-aged resident is often related to neurologic diseases, traumatic injury from a work or a motor vehicle accident, or cardiovascular disease, such as strokes and coronary artery disease. Like the younger adult, the middle-aged resident has special needs and

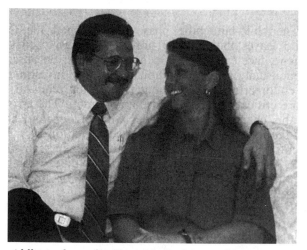

Figure 3–3. A middle-aged couple. (From Medical-Surgical Nursing: A Nursing Process Approach, *2nd ed. (p. 54), by D.D. Ignatavicius, M.L. Workman, & M.A. Mishler, 1995, Philadelphia: W.B. Saunders. Reprinted with permission.)*

may feel isolated or different from many elderly nursing home residents who may be cognitively impaired and physically debilitated. Some middle-aged residents are able to undergo rehabilitation for their health problem and be discharged to home or another level of care, such as a group home.

Assessment of the Newly Admitted Nursing Home Resident

ASSESSMENT PRIOR TO ADMISSION

Assessment of the resident entering a nursing home may begin before admission. The admissions director or social worker relays essential information to the nurse regarding medical diagnosis; physician; level of care; need for equipment, such as oxygen; functional and cognitive ability; and third-party information.

If the resident is admitted from another facility, such as a hospital, the discharge summary, transfer summary, plan of care, and assessment data, such as laboratory test results, should accompany the resident. If the attending physician who cared for the person in the hospital will continue care in the nursing home, admitting physician's orders may also accompany the resident on admission. According to recent standards of the Joint Commission on Accreditation of Healthcare Organizations (JCAHO), a nurse from the transferring facility must also call the nursing home to promote a "seamless" flow of information between health care agencies.

The new resident should also have a mental identification (ID) screening before or on admission. Known as PASARR (Preadmission Screening/Annual Resident Review), this federally mandated assessment form is usually completed by the social worker from the transferring facility before admission or at the time of admission. If the resident is admitted directly from the community, the geriatric evaluation service (GES), social worker, or physician may complete the form. The purpose of the screening tool is to identify residents who have, or are at risk for, mental illness or mental retardation. If the screening is "positive" for either of these health problems, placement for the resident needs to be reevaluated to ensure that the resident is in the best type of facility for his or her mental health problem. A sample PASARR form is found in Appendix B.

INITIAL RESIDENT ASSESSMENT

Nursing Assessment

The nurse performs a history, where additional psychosocial information can be obtained, and a head-to-toe physical assessment on the resident. The family or significant other is also interviewed to collect information as well as to identify family concerns. The nurse can offer reassurance at this time to help ease the transition into the facility as well as to help the family resolve the guilt that typically exists.

The nursing assessment database is completed during the first 24 hours after admission. Currently, there is no standard form used among nursing homes for this purpose.

Minimum Data Set

Because the focus of care in a nursing home is interdisciplinary, the federal government, as part of the Omnibus Budget Reconciliation Act of 1987, mandated that a standardized interdisciplinary assessment tool be used across the country. In 1990, the first version of the Minimum Data Set (MDS) and its accompanying resident assessment protocols (RAPs) were introduced. The MDS must be completed within the first 14 days after admission or when there is a significant change in the resident's condition. Each discipline assesses its related component. For example, the section on psychosocial well-being is completed by the social worker, the section on oral/nutritional status is completed by the dietitian, and the section on activity pursuit patterns is completed by the activity therapist. Most of the MDS is assessed by the nurse, either an LPN or RN. However, the RN who coordinates the comprehensive assessment must sign the MDS. A quarterly update must also be completed for each resident.

On January 1, 1996, a new version of the MDS (called the 2.0 version) was implemented. The new version is not dramatically different but rather presents more specific questions in some of the assessment areas. A sample of a completed MDS 2.0 is found in Appendix C.

The RAPs simply identify 18 resident health problem areas, such as falls, pressure ulcers, and delirium, that may be appropriate, based on responses to the MDS tool. Each applicable resident problem must be addressed, either as part of the care plan or elsewhere in the resident's medical record. A sample of these forms is also located in Appendix C.

In addition to the initial nursing assessment tool and the MDS, additional assessments that focus on specific health areas may be required by the nursing home. For example, some nursing homes have adopted a functional assessment tool to critically assess the resident's mobility and ability to carry out activities of daily living (ADLs). Others require that a mental status assessment using a specified tool must be completed. These additional assessment tools are discussed in the next chapter.

Focused Assessments

In the hospital setting, where the patients are acutely ill and the ratio of licensed staff is higher than in a nursing home, head-to-toe physical assessments are performed on every patient at least once per shift. In the nursing home, this practice is not feasible. However, in lieu of regular physical assessments, the nurse is responsible for following up on resident complaints or observations made by unlicensed staff, especially geriatric nursing assistants (GNAs).

A focused assessment is specifically based on a diagnosis, symptom/sign, or body system. For example, if the GNA reports that a resident has a cough, there may be a tendency for the nurse to check the medication administration record (MAR) for a cough medication to be administered as circumstances require (PRN), rather than first take the time to perform a respiratory physical assessment. This practice is especially likely to occur if the nurse is familiar with the resident or has a time constraint.

Although the nursing home population is generally considered to be more medically "stable" than patients in a hospital, nursing home residents are sicker today than in previous times as a result of earlier hospital discharges. This fact, added to the increasingly advanced age in the nursing home population, makes it even more important for nurses to refine and use their assessment skills. Chapter 6 discusses focused assessments for selected acute illnesses and health emergencies.

Transfers to Other Health Care Settings

In addition to conducting admission and ongoing assessments, the nurse assesses the resident and documents findings upon temporary or permanent discharge from the facility. If the resident is transferred to the hospital for evaluation or admission, most nursing homes require completion of a transfer summary that highlights the resident's current health status. In addition, it is often very helpful to the receiving unit to have the plan of care, history and physical examination record, and progress notes. The entire record should not accompany the resident.

CHAPTER HIGHLIGHTS

Physiologic changes associated with aging can be generally characterized as tissue degeneration and losses in tissue elasticity; these changes predispose the elderly to a variety of acute and chronic illnesses.

Many "normal" values for laboratory tests are affected by aging; these include hematocrit and lymphocyte count, which decrease with aging.

Psychosocial changes associated with the aging process include losses as well as gains in new roles.

An increasing number of young and middle-aged adults are admitted to nursing homes because they are surviving acute and chronic health problems; many of these residents feel isolated in a nursing home that has a majority of older residents.

The Preadmission Screening/Annual Resident Review (PASARR) and Minimum Data Set (MDS) are part of the assessment records that must be completed on admission to a nursing home

REFERENCES AND READINGS

Anderson, M.A., & Braun, J.V. (1995). *Caring for the elderly client.* Philadelphia: F.A. Davis.
Burbank, P.M. (1992). An exploratory study: Assessing the meaning of life among older adult clients. *Journal of Gerontological Nursing, 18*(9), 19–28.
Ebersole, P., & Hess, P. (1994). *Toward healthy aging.* St. Louis: Mosby.
Eliopoulos, C. (1990). *Health assessment of the older adult.* Redwood City, CA: Addison-Wesley.
Garner, B.C. (1989). Guide to changing lab values in elders. *Geriatric Nursing, 21*(3), 144–145.
Giger, J.N., & Davidhizar, R.E. (1995). *Transcultural nursing: Assessment and intervention.* St. Louis: Mosby Year Book.
Heriot, C.S. (1992). Spirituality and aging. *Holistic Nursing Practice, 7*(1), 22–31.
Ignatavicius, D.D., Workman, M.L., & Mishler, M.M. (1995). *Medical-surgical nursing: A nursing process approach.* Philadelphia: W.B. Saunders.
Jarvis, C. (1996). *Physical examination and health assessment.* Philadelphia: W.B. Saunders.
Koenig, H. (1987). Religion and well-being in later life. In *Proceedings of the Third Congress of the International Psychogeriatric Association.* Chicago: International Psychogeriatric Association.
Lee, C., Barrett, A., & Ignatavicius, D. (1996). *Fluids and electrolytes: A practical approach.* Philadelphia: F.A. Davis.
Mezey, M.D., Rauckhorst, L.H., & Stokes, S.A. (1993). *Health assessment of the older adult.* New York: Springer.
Tietz, N.W. (1995). *Clinical guide to laboratory tests* (3rd ed.). Philadelphia: W.B. Saunders.

DISCUSSION QUESTIONS TO PROMOTE CRITICAL THINKING

1. What nursing interventions are appropriate when caring for an elderly client with thin, fragile skin?

2. What nursing interventions are appropriate for the elderly client with deceased sensory function (presbyopia and presbycusis)?

3. In the nursing home setting, what interventions are appropriate for elderly clients as a result of bladder and bowel changes?

4

Common Health Problems of Residents in Nursing Homes

OUTLINE

Falls
Pressure Ulcers
Urinary Incontinence
Cognitive Dysfunction
Malnutrition
Constipation
Diarrhea

OBJECTIVES

- Identify factors that place a resident at risk for falls
- Describe nursing assessment and interventions for the resident who experiences a fall
- List two assessment tools commonly used to assess a resident's risk for pressure ulcers
- Identify the four stages of pressure ulcers
- Define five types of chronic urinary incontinence and how they are managed
- Differentiate three common mental health problems experienced by the elderly—delirium, depression, and dementia
- Describe nursing interventions for residents experiencing delirium, depression, and/or dementia

- Describe how to perform a nutritional assessment for a resident in a nursing home
- Discuss the nurse's role in caring for the resident receiving enteral and parenteral nutrition
- Identify nursing interventions for prevention and management or constipation and diarrhea

Most residents in nursing homes experience one or more health problems that are not necessarily related to their medical diagnoses. Most of these common problems occur with residents over 65 years of age, but are not limited to this age group.

Falls

The National Institute on Aging (1990) estimates that about one-third of all elderly people fall at least once. Falls in the community elderly are usually not reported. The incidence of falls in the institutionalized elderly is between 40 percent and 50 percent.

Falls are an important health care concern because they can result in both physical and emotional damage. Fractures, head injury, and soft tissue trauma are common examples of physical impairment. These injuries often lead to a general decline in health, or even death. The psychological fear ("fallaphobia") associated with falls can also be devastating. Elders who have a history of one or more falls are especially vulnerable to this emotional response (Tideiksaar, 1993).

FACTORS CONTRIBUTING TO FALLS

The contributing factors that predispose an elderly person to fall can be divided into two broad areas—physiologic changes associated with the aging process and other biopsychosocial factors (Table 4–1).

Physiologic Changes That Contribute to Falls

As a person ages, the skeleton loses some bone mass. Osteoporosis occurs when bone loss is severe, leaving the bones porous and brittle. Kyphosis of the osteoporotic thoracic spine changes the elderly person's gait and

Table 4–1. **Factors Contributing to Falls in Nursing Homes**

Physiologic Changes Associated with Aging
Osteoporosis (especially in women)
Kyphosis (stooped posture)
Gait changes
Decreased balance and coordination
Diminished peripheral sensation
Weak bladder
Need for increased lighting and/or vision impairment
Muscle atrophy
Decreased reaction time

Other Factors
Acute illness, such as infection
Chronic illness, such as arthritis
Impaired mobility, such as that due to stroke or Parkinson's disease
Pain
Cognitive impairment, such as dementia
Drugs that cause hypotension or sedation
Fatigue
"Sundowning"
History of one or more falls
Environmental hazards, such as wet floors
Lack of necessary assistive or ambulatory devices
Lack of supervision
Relocation trauma

center of gravity, affecting balance and coordination. As discussed in Chapter 3, women are more likely than men to experience osteoporosis. In some cases, the bone may actually break *before* the fall. In addition to the risk from osteoporosis, decreased reaction time, diminished coordination ability and balance, and muscle atrophy contribute to the likelihood of falls.

Decreased peripheral sensation resulting from slower circulation may hinder a person's ability to feel where feet are placed when ambulating. Steps are particularly hazardous.

The bladder of an elder has diminished capacity, leading to urinary frequency. As a result, nocturia (voiding during the night) is very common among the elderly. During the night, the elder may attempt to reach the bathroom and fall, often because he or she becomes temporarily disoriented. In some cases, the individual in a nursing home or hospital doesn't want to "bother" the staff and gets out of bed without calling for assistance.

An elderly person also requires as much as 50 percent more light than younger adults to see clearly at night. The night staff may typically lower the lights at night to encourage sleep, not realizing that the elderly person needs *more* light at night when ambulating.

Other Factors Contributing to Falls

In a nursing home, there are many additional factors that place the resident at a high risk for falling. Some of these factors are related to the resident's condition, while others are related to the resident's environment.

Physical and Mental Conditions

Residents in nursing homes are at high risk for falling because they often have acute and chronic illnesses that compromise their ability to move. For example, residents with strokes have one-sided weakness or paralysis; residents with Parkinson's disease are stiff and have a shuffling gait. Pain can also limit mobility, especially for residents with arthritis or other musculoskeletal dysfunction.

Residents with cognitive impairments, such as dementia, are also at risk for falls because they do not understand the need to call for assistance when getting out of bed or walking.

Drug therapy alone can create problems that make residents likely to fall. For instance, most antihypertensive medications can cause dizziness or syncope (blackouts) from orthostatic hypotension and bradycardia (pulse below 60 bpm). When the individual moves from a lying or sitting position to stand, the systolic and/or diastolic blood pressure drops by between 10 and 20 mm Hg and the resident becomes dizzy and weak. Other commonly used drugs such as Sinemet (antiparkinsonian drug) and haloperidol (Haldol; antipsychotic drug) cause severe orthostatic hypotension, and sedation as well. When residents need opioid analgesia (narcotics) for acute pain, blood pressure may also decrease.

Most studies of falls show that when residents are tired, especially in the evening, they are prone to falls. Fatigue, combined with "sundowning," in which the demented resident becomes increasingly disoriented, predisposes an elderly resident to falls around bedtime. And residents with a history of at least one fall are likely to experience another fall.

Environmental Factors

For the newly admitted resident in a nursing home, the unfamiliarity of the environment can contribute to falling. Maintaining a hazard-free environment is crucial in fall prevention. The staff must be aware of potential hazards and remove them as soon as possible. Examples of hazards include wet or highly polished floors, clutter in the resident's room or hall, and rearranged furniture.

In addition, staff must ensure that the resident has access to the call light as well as his or her customary sensory aids, such as glasses, hearing aids, and ambulatory devices (walkers and canes). The resident should wear proper shoes with leather or rubber soles that provide adequate support. The staff must also be trained in proper transfer techniques and be able to assist the resident safely during ambulation.

Supervision of residents is essential. Because most falls in nursing homes occur at the bedside, periodic rounds of residents in their rooms or in group settings, such as the activity room, are essential.

PREVENTION OF FALLS

Risk Assessment

The first step in preventing falls is to determine who is most at risk for falling. A number of fall assessment tools are available, but the Minimum Data Set also helps determine who is at the greatest risk of falls (Appendix C). Many facilities identify the residents at highest risk and place a sign or "falling star" emblem at the bedside to remind all staff which residents need special attention.

Another step in fall prevention is to study the fall pattern within the nursing home. While the literature describes typical times and locations for falls (Baker & Harvey 1985; Tinetti & Speechley, 1990), each facility has its own characteristics. For example, when the author was director of nursing at a large retirement center, the most frequent time of falls was *not* during the daytime as the literature indicated. Instead, based on the previous year's incident reports, most falls in the skilled nursing facility occurred between 4 PM and 9 PM.

On further evaluation, the staff felt that decreased staffing in the period from 3 PM to 11 PM, resident fatigue, and the scheduling of dinner breaks for the nursing assistants all contributed to the evening fall pattern. New action steps for fall prevention then included an increased staffing ratio, an increased number of residents who ate in the dining room with group supervision, and a more appropriate dinner break schedule for the staff. On follow-up evaluation, the incidence of falls decreased as a result of these action steps (see Chapter 14 for more discussion of quality improvement).

Interventions for Preventing Falls

After identifying which residents are at the highest risk for falls and examining the fall pattern in the facility, interventions to provide a safe, hazard-free environment must be implemented. Staff members must be educated about avoiding clutter, cleaning spills immediately, and providing ambulatory aids, including hand rails in the hallways and bathrooms. More facilities are currently using carpet on their floors to help "cushion" falls. Frequent supervised toileting can help reduce falls as well.

In the past, side rails and physical restraints were used with the intent of fall prevention, but these measures inhibit a resident's ability to move and are no longer acceptable practice for fall prevention (see later discussion of restraints in this chapter under "Cognitive Dysfunction"). Mattresses placed on the floor or low cots, such as futons, can prevent injuries due to falling out of bed. Less restrictive devices like the "Lap Buddy" are preferred over vest restraints.

Another important intervention for preventing falls is to maintain mobility of the residents through an aggressive rehabilitative and restorative therapy program. In some facilities, restorative or physical therapy aides ambulate residents, help with bed-to-chair transfers, and perform range-of-motion exercises to keep residents as mobile as possible.

For residents who fall, a nursing assessment to determine contributing factors is also important. For instance, the resident may be taking a medication whose side effects contributed to the fall. The physician may need to discontinue the drug or lower its dosage. Or the resident may have forgotten to use the call light to summon assistance before getting out of a chair. In this case, the staff must emphasize to the resident the necessity of using the call light before ambulating.

Despite all these interventions, some residents experience multiple falls. For these residents, more aggressive methods for fall prevention are necessary. Some families desire one-to-one supervision for their loved one and therefore may employ a sitter to supervise the resident. For many residents, though, this intervention is too costly.

An alternative to continuous direct supervision is a mechanical device to alert the staff when the resident begins to move without assistance. One popular pressure-sensitive device is placed over the mattress and activates an alarm when the resident begins to get out of bed.

ASSESSMENT AND INTERVENTIONS FOR RESIDENTS EXPERIENCING FALLS

No matter what specific fall prevention and education measures are used in nursing homes, some residents continue to fall. When a fall occurs, the nurse performs a resident assessment to determine not only the cause of the fall but also the physical condition of the resident (Table 4–2).

Table 4–2. **Assessment of the Resident Experiencing a Fall**

- Check the airway and ease of breathing; assess respiratory rate and quality.
- Perform a neurologic assessment
  □ Assess level of consciousness (alert, drowsy, or not conscious).
  □ Ask the resident to move all extemities, if possible.
  □ Ask the resident, if he or she is able to communicate, whether pain or other unusual sensation is present; if pain is present, determine location.
  □ Check blood pressure and pulse.
  □ Check pupils for reaction to light.
- Check all extremities for pain, alignment, and symmetry.
- Assess skin for intactness, bruising, and swelling.
- Compare all assessment findings with baseline status before the fall.
- Document all assessment findings in the medical record.

Although the most important aspect to be assessed following trauma is airway, falls rarely affect a resident's ability to breathe. Most residents are very anxious, however, and may hyperventilate. The nurse should reassure the resident in a calm tone of voice.

The next step is to assess level of consciousness (LOC). If the resident has a severe head injury, a decreasing LOC is indicative of increased intracranial pressure, a life-threatening problem. The Glasgow Coma Scale is a tool frequently used to evaluate LOC (Fig. 4–1). Neurologic assessment should also be carried out by other measures, such as vital signs, ability to move, and pupillary response.

Because hip fracture is a result or cause of falls, special attention should be given to both lower extremities. Pain in the groin or knee, leg rotation, and leg shortening are classic signs and symptoms of a hip fracture.

GLASGOW COMA SCALE*

Eye Opening

Spontaneous	4
To sound	3
To pain	2
Never	1

Motor Response

Obeys commands	6
Localizes pain	5
Normal flexion (withdrawal)	4
Abnormal flexion	3
Extension	2
Nil	1

Verbal Response

Oriented	5
Confused conversation	4
Inappropriate words	3
Incomprehensible sounds	2
None	1

* The highest possible score is 15

Figure 4–1. The Glasgow Coma Scale. From *Medical-Surgical Nursing: A Nursing Process Approach* (p. 103), by D. D. Ignatavicius, M. L. Workman, and M. A. Mishler, 1995, Philadelphia: W. B. Saunders. Reprinted with permission.

Not all of these manifestations need to be present for a hip fracture to be suspected. If there is any question of possible injury, the resident needs a thorough evaluation, including x-rays.

Following any fall, the staff continues to monitor the resident for significant changes in physical or mental condition. The trauma of the fall can contribute to acute confusion, known as delirium, discussed later in this chapter.

Pressure Ulcers

Pressure ulcers, sometimes called decubitus ulcers or pressure sores, are a major concern for elderly populations in health care facilities as well as home settings. Among residents in nursing homes, the prevalence of pressure ulcers was found to be 23 percent (Young, 1989). Many residents with pressure ulcers acquire them in the hospital or home setting before admission to the nursing home.

Like falls, pressure ulcers often lead to negative outcomes for the resident, as well as malpractice claims against the nursing home and its staff. Some of the most common complications of pressure ulcers include pain; cellulitis (tissue inflammation and infection); and sepsis, which can lead to dehydration, septic shock, and even death.

FACTORS CONTRIBUTING TO FORMATION OF PRESSURE ULCERS

A number of risk factors predispose a person to pressure ulcers. These factors can be broadly categorized as physiologic changes associated with aging (for elderly residents) and other biopsychosocial factors.

Physiologic Changes Associated with Aging

Although the elderly population is not the only group in a nursing home that develops pressure ulcers, physiologic changes associated with the aging process predispose an elderly person more than a younger person to this health problem. These changes include thinner skin, diminished subcutaneous tissue, decreased mobility, and decreased skin pressure receptors. When an elderly person develops an ulcer, healing time is increased due to decreased blood supply to the skin and its underlying tissues. Some wounds in the elderly can take as much as 100 days to heal, at a cost estimated to be over $20,000 (Ebersole & Hess, 1994).

Other Factors Contributing to Pressure Ulcers

As in the case of falls, contributing factors for pressure ulcer development stem from the resident's physical and mental condition, as well as from the environment.

Physical and Mental Condition

Pressure ulcers typically occur over bony prominences, and therefore thin, frail elderly individuals are at a very high risk. Other groups at risk include those residents who are on chronic corticosteroid therapy (making skin "thinner"); those with poor nutritional status, hypoalbuminemia (decreased serum albumin), and anemia; those who cannot move independently, either because of a health problem or drug-induced sedation; those with impaired sensation, such as the spinal cord–injured resident; and those who are incontinent.

Environmental Factors

When residents are not moved frequently, or remain wet from urine or perspiration, they are very prone to skin breakdown. Therefore, the staff in a nursing home must be well educated about the importance of keeping residents dry and of turning and repositioning them without shearing the skin.

If residents are restrained, either with a physical restraint such as a Posey vest or by medication (chemical restraint), they are unable to freely move and can readily develop a pressure ulcer. By federal law, residents in a nursing home have the right to be free of both types of restraints.

PREVENTION OF PRESSURE ULCERS

Risk Assessment

The first step in preventing pressure ulcers is to identify the individuals most at risk. After careful review and analysis of a large body of research literature, the Agency for Health Care Policy and Research (AHCPR) recommends one of two tools that, for predicting pressure ulcer development, give a more in-depth skin assessment than the Minimum Data Set. These are the Norton Scale and the Braden Scale (Panel for the Prediction and Prevention of Pressure Ulcers in Adults, 1992).

The Norton Scale rates the resident's physical condition, mental condition, activity, mobility, and incontinence. The resident can score from a low of 5 (very high risk of pressure ulcers) to 20 (lowered risk).

The Braden Scale for predicting pressure sore risk is based on measures of sensory perception, moisture, activity, mobility, nutrition, and friction and shear potential (Fig. 4–2). Like the Norton Scale, the lower scores correlate with the highest risk. Both assessment tools are easy to use and take 2 to 3 minutes to complete. Both tools can be used for baseline assessment as well as for ongoing assessment when the resident's overall condition changes.

Interventions for Preventing Pressure Ulcers

The interventions described in Table 4–3 are part of the clinical practice guidelines advocated by the AHCPR. They include both prevention and

Client's Name _____ Evaluator's Name _____ Date of Assessment

	1	2	3	4		
Sensory perception Ability to respond meaningfully to pressure-related discomfort	**1. Completely limited** Unresponsive (does not moan, flinch, or grasp) to painful stimuli because of diminished level of consciousness or sedation OR limited ability to feel pain over most of body surface	**2. Very limited** Responds only to painful stimuli; cannot communicate discomfort except by moaning or restlessness OR has a sensory impairment that limits the ability to feel pain or discomfort over 1/2 of the body	**3. Slightly limited** Responds to verbal commands but cannot always communicate discomfort or need to be turned OR has some sensory impairment that limits ability to feel pain or discomfort in 1 or 2 extremities	**4. No impairment** Responds to verbal commands; has no sensory deficit that would limit ability to feel or voice pain or discomfort		
Moisture Degree to which skin is exposed to moisture	**1. Completely moist** Skin is kept moist almost constantly by perspiration, urine; dampness is detected every time the client is moved or turned	**2. Moist** Skin is often but not always moist; linen must be changed at least once a shift	**3. Occasionally moist** Skin is occasionally moist, requiring an extra linen change approximately once a day	**4. Rarely moist** Skin is usually dry; linen requires changing only at routine intervals		
Activity Degree of physical activity	**1. Bedfast** Confined to bed	**2. Chairfast** Ability to walk severely limited or nonexistent; cannot bear own weight and must be assisted into chair or wheelchair	**3. Walks occasionally** Walks occasionally during the day but for very short distances, with or without assistance; spends the majority of each shift in bed or chair	**4. Walks frequently** Walks outside the room at least twice a day and inside the room at least once every 2 hours during walking hours		
Mobility Ability to change or control body position	**1. Completely immobile** Does not make even slight changes in body or extremity position without assistance	**2. Very limited** Makes occasional slight changes in body or extremity position but unable to make frequent or significant changes independently	**3. Slightly limited** Makes frequent though slight changes in body or extremity position independently	**4. No limitations** Makes major and frequent changes in position without assistance		
Nutrition Usual food intake pattern	**1. Very poor** Never eats a complete meal; rarely eats more than 1/3 of any food offered; eats 2 servings or less of protein (meat or dairy products) per day; takes fluids poorly; does not take a liquid dietary supplement OR is NPO or maintained on clear liquids or IV for more than 5 days	**2. Probably inadequate** Rarely eats a complete meal and generally eats only about 1/2 of any food offered; protein intake includes only 3 servings of meat or dairy products per day; occasionally will take a dietary supplement OR receives less than optimal amount of liquid diet or tube feeding	**3. Adequate** Eats over half of most meals; eats a total of 4 servings of protein (meat, dairy products) each day; occasionally will refuse a meal, but will usually take a supplement if offered OR is receiving tube feeding or total parenteral nutrition, which probably meets most nutritional needs	**4. Excellent** Eats most of every meal; never refuses a meal; usually eats a total of 4 or more servings of meat and dairy products; occasionally eats between meals; does not require supplementation		
Friction and shear	**1. Problem** Requires moderate to maximum assistance in moving; complete lifting without sliding against sheets is impossible; frequently slides down in bed or chair, requiring frequent repositioning with maximum assistance; spasticity, contractures, or agitation leads to almost constant friction	**2. Potential problem** Moves feebly or requires minimum assistance; during a move, skin probably slides to some extent against sheets, chair, restraints, or other devices; maintains relatively good position in chair or bed most of the time but occasionally slides down	**3. No apparent problem** Moves in bed and in chair independently and has sufficient muscle strength to lift up completely during move; maintains good position in bed or chair at all times			

Total score _____

Figure 4-2. The Braden Scale for predicting pressure ulcer development.

Table 4–3. **Interventions for Prevention of Pressure Ulcers**

Risk Assessment Tools and Risk Factors
- Identify at-risk individuals and the factors placing them at risk.

Skin Care and Early Treatment
- Inspect skin daily, paying special attention to bony prominences; document findings.
- Clean soiled skin promptly, using a mild cleansing agent that minimizes skin irritation and dryness; avoid friction during cleansing.
- Minimize factors that can cause skin to dry, such as exposure to cold or low humidity; treat dry skin with moisturizers.
- Avoid massage over bony prominences.
- For incontinent residents, use underpads or briefs that absorb moisture and keep skin dry; use topical moisture barriers.
- Prevent skin injury due to friction and shearing by proper positioning, transferring, and turning techniques.
- Maintain adequate nutrition, especially a high intake of protein and calories.
- Improve or maintain mobility and activity level to the extent possible.
- Monitor the results of interventions and document according to facility policy.

Mechanical Loading and Support Surfaces
- Reposition all bed bound residents *at least* every 2 hours, using a written turning schedule if necessary.
- For bed bound residents, use positioning devices and pressure-relieving devices, such as pillows and foam wedges; keep bony prominences from direct contact with one another.
- Keep heels off of the bed at all times, using devices that totally relieve pressure; do not use donut-type devices.
- When the resident is side-lying, avoid positioning him or her directly on the trochanter.
- Maintain the head of the bed at the lowest possible degree of elevation to prevent sacral pressure; limit the amount of time the head of the bed is elevated.
- Use lifting devices, such as a trapeze or lift sheet, to move (rather than drag) the resident in bed.
- For high-risk residents, use pressure-reducing devices such as foam, alternating air, gel, or water mattresses.
- For residents in a chair or wheelchair, reposition every hour; if possible, teach the resident to shift weight every 15 minutes.

Education
- Provide organized, structured education about prevention of pressure ulcers for all levels of health care providers, including residents and their families or other caregivers.

Adapted from Agency on Health Care Policy and Research, *Pressure Ulcers in Adults: Prediction and Prevention* (1992).

early treatment for skin problems. As seen in the table, the best intervention for prevention and management of stage I pressure areas is preventing further pressure by turning and repositioning. Although the traditional turn schedule has been at least every 2 hours, research suggests that elderly clients need to be turned and repositioned at least every 1½ hours. The skin should be inspected each time the resident is turned.

Pressure-relieving support surfaces are also helpful in relieving pressure, especially on heels. A study by De Keyser et al. (1994) found that regular bed pillows were more effective than any commercial heel protective device in reducing pressure on the heels.

In addition to the interventions included in Table 4–3, the AHCPR recommmends that the incidence of pressure ulcers can be reduced through structured, comprehensive, interdisciplinary educational programs for staff members who provide resident care.

ASSESSMENT OF RESIDENTS WITH PRESSURE ULCERS

If a resident develops a pressure ulcer, accurate nursing assessment is essential for planning the appropriate interventions. Assessment includes observation, palpation, and measurement of the ulcer and surrounding tissue.

Observation of Pressure Ulcers

The nurse observes the affected area to determine if the skin is intact. The area may only be reddened with skin intact. If the skin is broken, the color of the wound is assessed, as well as the color and condition of the skin around the wound. If the area around the wound is reddened, cellulitis (tissue inflammation and infection) may be present. This indicates a need for systemic treatment in addition to local wound care.

The wound is also observed for drainage. The color, consistency, and odor of the drainage, if present, needs to be recorded and reported to the physician. The nurse also assesses the depth of the wound—by visual inspection as well as actual measurement, described later. Some wounds are deep enough to expose muscle or bone.

Palpation of Pressure Ulcers

Following observation, the nurse palpates the skin around an open area or touches an intact, reddened pressure area to assess warmth. An area that is warmer than skin elsewhere on the body indicates inflammation and possibly infection. In addition to gauging temperature, the texture of the skin needs to be determined. A soft, "mushy" texture over areas of prolonged pressure indicates dead tissue under the skin. The outer skin may be intact, but the tissue underneath may be necrotic.

Measurement of Pressure Ulcers

The reddened area or open wound must be measured—both in diameter and depth (for open areas). Disposable measuring devices are available for this purpose. The nurse also takes a sterile gloved hand or cotton swab and *gently* feels under the surrounding skin for fistulas, or "tunnels." If these are present, the ulcer has undermined adjacent tissue, and such a finding usually indicates infection.

Staging of Pressure Ulcers

Selecting the proper treatment for a pressure ulcer depends on a number of variables, including the depth and involvement of tissue, the presence of drainage, and the presence of local or systemic infection. One way to classify pressure ulcers is by using a staging system, stage I through stage IV.

According to the AHCPR guidelines, the skin is intact with a stage I ulcer. The pressure area is reddened and not blanchable, meaning that pressing the area with a finger does not change the color of the lesion. Higher level ulcers (stages II through IV) involve open wounds. Stage II ulcers, for example, have loss of partial skin thickness involving the epidermis and/or dermis layers. These ulcers are sometimes referred to as superficial and can appear as blisters, abrasions, or shallow craters.

Stage III ulcers have full-thickness skin loss involving damage to, or necrosis of, subcutaneous tissue; they can extend into, but not through, underlying fascia. These ulcers appear as deep craters with or without undermining of adjacent tissue.

Stage IV ulcers involve deep destruction of tissue through muscle, bone, or supporting structures. Undermining may also be present.

There are three additional points about staging:

1. Stage I pressure areas are more difficult to assess on dark-skinned individuals.
2. The presence of black eschar (tough, leathery necrotic tissue) prevents accurate staging until the eschar is removed.
3. After healing, the stage remains the same.

The Red-Yellow-Black System for Classifying Wounds

In an attempt to develop a simpler system for classifying wounds, including pressure ulcers, a classification based on wound color was introduced from Europe into the United States in 1988. The red-yellow-black (RYB) system is used as an adjunct to the traditional staging system for open wounds and helps to determine the correct treatment plan (Krasner, 1995).

Wounds can be red, yellow, or black, or a mixture of these colors. These colors reflect the stages of the healing process or suggest that the wound is not healing.

Red Wounds

Red wounds reflect the inflammatory phase of tissue healing. In the first 72 hours after wound development, the wound becomes reddened and swollen, a characteristic of the reaction phase. Over the next several weeks, granulation tissue develops, in which tissue regenerates. The remodeling phase of the healing process allows the scar tissue to reorganize and gain strength over a period of months.

Yellow Wounds

Yellow wounds often suggest infection, either local (contained within the wound) or systemic (throughout other body tissues). Drainage from yellow wounds may be green or cream-colored (pus) and may contain an accumulation of bacteria, white blood cells, and cellular debris.

Black Wounds

Like yellow wounds, black wounds are not involved in the healing process. Devitalized, dried collagen, called eschar, can be black, gray, brown, or tan. It is thick and leathery in texture, and must be removed (debrided) before healing can begin. Debridement must be performed cautiously in patients with leukopenia or vascular disease.

INTERVENTIONS FOR RESIDENTS WITH PRESSURE ULCERS

Management of pressure ulcers depends on many factors, including the stage of the wound and the presence of infection. Wounds with dead tissue (black wounds) must be debrided before healing can occur. A number of debridement methods are available, employing enzymatic topical agents, surgical debridement, hydrophilic beads, and wet-to-damp gauze dressings. Once the area is debrided, the wound cleansing and dressing technique is changed to promote protection during the healing process.

The traditional dressing material for ulcers has been cotton gauze, used either for protection during healing or debridement. When a physician or enterostomal therapist prescribes continuous dry dressings, the purpose is usually to absorb drainage and to protect the damaged tissue. If the order is for wet-to-dry or wet-to-damp dressings, the gauze is applied wet, usually with saline, and removed when it is either dry or damp to debride the wound. Povidone-iodine (Betadine) should not be used on pressure ulcers because it destroys granulation tissue. Dakin's solution or another similar product may be used as an antiseptic. All gauze dressings must be changed when "strike-through" occurs—when the drainage can be seen on the outer layer of the dressing (Cuzzell, 1995).

Two newer types of synthetic dressings are the hydrophobics and the hydrophilics. *Hydrophobic* materials are nonabsorbent and waterproof, and are used when the wound has minimal or no drainage (red wounds). The purpose of this type of dressing is to protect the wound while it is healing. Examples are DuoDerm and Tegaderm. *Hydrophilic* materials are absorbent and are used to draw excessive drainage away from the wound (yellow wounds). Examples are Kaltostat and Sorbsan (alginates).

Synthetic dressings should be changed when accumulation of exudate (drainage) causes the seal to break and leakage occurs.

Regardless of the type of dressing, all wounds should be cleaned with saline or an antibacterial solution like Hibiclens before new dressings are reapplied.

In addition to wound management, interventions to help heal pressure ulcers include increased nutrition, particularly increased protein, iron, zinc, and vitamin C. Dietary supplements as well as drug therapy can be used to increase the intake of those nutrients. Zinc has recently been found to have a key role in tissue healing (Lee, Barrett, & Ignatavicius, 1996). Additional interventions for meeting the nutritional needs of nursing home residents are discussed later in this chapter under the health problem "Undernutrition."

Urinary Incontinence

Urinary incontinence, the involuntary loss of urine from the urinary tract, is *not* a normal physiologic change associated with aging. However, some physiologic changes can predispose an elderly individual to this very common health problem. The National Institutes of Health estimate that at least half of all nursing home residents and 3 out of every 10 elders who live in the community are incontinent (National Institutes of Health Urinary Incontinence in Adults, Consensus Conference: 1990).

Left untreated, urinary incontinence can have a devastating impact, both physically and psychologically. The two major physical complications of incontinence are skin breakdown and urinary tract infection (UTI). Falls can also result from incontinence because some elders stand, void, then slip in their urine.

Urinary incontinence can be very distressing and embarassing for anyone, regardless of age. The incontinent individual usually withdraws from social interaction for fear of having an "accident." The results can be social isolation and perhaps depression.

Urinary incontinence among residents in a nursing home is a very costly health problem in terms of supplies, linen, and human resources. Nursing homes devote the equivalent of two full-time staff members each day for care of urinary incontinence (Cella, 1988).

FACTORS CONTRIBUTING TO URINARY INCONTINENCE

Urinary incontinence affects people of all ages but is most often associated with the elderly population. Age-related changes, such as prostate enlargement in men, weakened pelvic floor muscles in women, decreased bladder capacity, and diminished bladder muscle contractions all predispose a resident to incontinence. Additionally, the characteristic nocturnal void-ing pattern means that older adults excrete most of their daily ingested fluid at night rather than during the day.

Urinary incontinence can occur suddenly (acute) or can progress slowly over years (chronic). Contributing factors other than age help to classify these broad types and identify more specific types of chronic uri-nary incontinence.

TYPES OF URINARY INCONTINENCE

Acute Urinary Incontinence

Acute incontinence, also called transient incontinence, occurs as a result of a number of factors. One way to summarize the common causes of acute urinary incontinence is by remembering the term DRIP:

    D = Delirium, drugs, diabetes
    R = Restricted mobility, urinary retention
    I = Infection, impaction
    P = Psychological problems, prescribed drugs, polyuria

Chronic Urinary Incontinence

Chronic urinary incontinence can be divided into five well-established types—stress, overflow, urge, functional, and mixed.

Stress Incontinence

Occurring primarily in women, stress incontinence is an involuntary loss of urine in small amounts (dribbling) when the pressure within the abdomen increases, such as during coughing, sneezing, laughing, lifting, and exercise. Contributing factors include obesity, aging, multiparity (mul-tiple childbirths), menopause (estrogen depletion), and surgical trauma.

Overflow Incontinence

Overflow incontinence primarily affects elderly men and is the involun-tary loss of urine in small amounts (dribbling) that occurs when the blad-der pressure exceeds the urethral pressure. The symptoms, which may be intermittent or continuous, result from a distended bladder. The most common cause of overflow incontinence is an enlarged prostate gland, which constricts the urethra and results in urinary retention. Other causes include medication, fecal impaction, and an atonic bladder muscle.

Medications that can contribute to overflow incontinence are anti-depressants, anticholinergics, antipsychotics, and muscle relaxants. All of these drugs cause urinary retention by preventing complete bladder emp-tying and promoting constipation.

Bladder muscle weakness leading to urinary retention is often caused by neurologic injury or disease, such as spinal cord injury, stroke, diabetes mellitus, and multiple sclerosis. The flaccid, neurogenic bladder caused by these conditions leads to inadequate bladder emptying.

Urge Incontinence

Urge incontinence is the most common type of incontinence for both elderly men and women. When the individual has the urge to urinate, he or she is unable to retain the urine before it leaks in moderate to large amounts. Common causes of this uninhibited bladder include stroke, dementia, and Parkinson's disease.

Functional Incontinence

In functional incontinence, the anatomy and physiology of the urinary tract is not affected. However, for a number of reasons, the individual is unable to go to the toilet or use the bedpan in a timely fashion. The resident may have impaired mobility due to arthritis, multiple sclerosis, or muscle weakness; or may have a cognitive dysfunction that prevents the person from moving to the appropriate place for elimination. In some cases, problems with the environment contribute to functional incontinence, such as a resident not knowing where the bathroom is located or not having a request for toileting answered promptly.

Mixed Incontinence

In the elderly population, it is not uncommon for a person to have several types of incontinence, often a combination of stress and urge incontinence.

PREVENTION OF URINARY INCONTINENCE

Prevention focuses on reducing the risk factors for incontinence when possible. For example, avoiding drugs that cause urinary retention is an important part of the prevention plan. Older adults and other residents at risk for urinary tract infection should be encouraged to drink adequate fluids daily—at least 2000 to 2500 mL per day, unless otherwise contraindicated (such as in cases of congestive heart or renal failure). Good bowel habits need to be promoted to prevent constipation, which could then lead to fecal impaction. Measures for prevention of constipation are discussed later in this chapter.

ASSESSMENT OF RESIDENTS
WITH URINARY INCONTINENCE

Nursing assessment of incontinence includes a thorough history to determine risk factors and documentation to ascertain the resident's voiding pattern. The nurse assesses for urinary retention by measuring intake and output, and palpating the abdomen for bladder distention. A rectal exam may reveal fecal impaction as a cause of the incontinence.

For residents who void but may retain residual urine, the physician may order a straight ("in-and-out") catheterization for residual urine within 10 to 15 minutes after spontaneous voiding. The normal postvoid residual amount is less than 100 to 150 mL. A urine specimen may be sent to the laboratory to analyze for bacterial growth, protein, and glucose.

INTERVENTIONS FOR RESIDENTS WITH URINARY INCONTINENCE

Interventions for incontinence depend on the type of incontinence and the age of the resident. For residents with acute or transient incontinence, removal or treatment of the cause is the most appropriate intervention. For example, a urinary tract infection may need antibiotic therapy; a drug promoting urinary retention may need to be discontinued; an impaction may need to be removed.

An assessment of the type of chronic incontinence present helps to determine the treatment plan. For some types of incontinence, individualized bladder retraining is possible. Bladder retraining helps to restore baseline voiding by scheduling the resident on a rigid toileting pattern. If the resident cannot void spontaneously, a catheterization schedule combined with the Credé maneuver (pressing over the bladder to facilitate emptying) may be useful, especially for overflow incontinence. Table 4–4 highlights the common interventions used to manage the resident with chronic incontinence.

Cognitive Dysfunction

Although an individual experiences many physiologic changes during the aging process, cognitive function does *not* change. An elderly person continues to have the capacity to learn but may take a little longer to learn new information. On the other hand, an elderly person is typically not able to adjust to environmental, health, and life changes as well as a younger person and therefore is predisposed to mental health problems, especially delirium and depression. In addition, some elders have a progressive cognitive impairment known as dementia. Delirium, depression, and dementia make up the 3Ds associated with mental health problems in the elderly.

DELIRIUM

Delirium (also called an acute confusional state) is an acute onset of cognitive dysfunction in which psychomotor, behavioral, and emotional

Table 4–4. **Interventions for Chronic Urinary Incontinence**

Type of Incontinence	Primary Interventions
Stress incontinence	Teach resident to practice Kegel exercises 2–3 times daily (contraction of pelvic floor muscles), if able.
	Wear protective pad inside underwear.
	If atrophic vaginitis is present, apply topical estrogen preparation to urethra daily.
	As a last resort, use alpha-adrenergic medications (e.g., Ditropan) to help retain urine.
Overflow incontinence	Identify, then treat or remove the cause.
	Avoid urine-retaining drugs, especially anticholinergics.
	If the cause is neurologic disease or trauma, place the resident on an intermittent catheterization schedule or Credé (pressing over bladder to facilitate emptying) schedule.
Urge incontinence	Toilet resident every 1–2 hours, based on usual voiding pattern; increase intervals to every 3–4 hours.
	Use bedside commode if resident is unable to reach bathroom.
Functional incontinence	Answer call light promptly.
	Mark the bathroom so that the resident can locate it easily.
	Toilet the resident every 1–2 hours.
	Consult with physical therapist to increase resident mobility.

responses, such as hallucinations and severe agitation, are common. The individual's recent memory is lost, and the sleep-wake cycle is disrupted.

The causes of delirium can be divided into systemic, mechanical, and psychosocial and/or environmental factors. Examples of *systemic* causes are surgery, drugs, infection, acute illness, endocrine or metabolic imbalances, dehydration, and pain. Women who experience a fractured hip are one of the most likely groups to have delirium. The pain of the fracture, the relocation into a hospital (*psychosocial* factor), and treatment (usually surgery) combine to cause acute confusion. The postoperative hip client may return from surgery screaming and attempting to climb over the side rails of the bed. The client is typically disoriented and confused, and is not aware of her surroundings.

Delirium is also commonly caused by medications, especially anticholinergic, cardiovascular, and analgesic drugs. Other causative factors include acute illness and infections, such as urinary tract infection. In some conditions, such as pneumonia and myocardial infarction, hypoxia (decreased oxygen to the brain) may cause acute confusion.

The major *mechanical* etiology of delirium is vascular disruption in the brain, usually caused by a cerebrovascular accident (CVA, or stroke).

Like other illnesses that decrease oxygen delivery to the brain, a CVA decreases blood flow to a part of the brain, often due to a clot. The result, then, is a diminished oxygen supply and subsequent acute confusion.

Whether the cause is organic (physical) or a response to stress, delirium is characteristically transient, meaning that it is short-term and usually resolves or improves in about 1 month or less.

Prevention of Delirium

Preventing delirium is not always possible, because some elderly residents experience many significant health or life changes. However, some preventive measures are helpful, such as avoiding drugs that are known to cause delirium and avoiding relocation, if possible. Other medication-related interventions to prevent delirium include:

- Reduce the number and amount of medications used in the elderly.
- Change one drug at a time, if a change is needed.
- Use low doses of medication and increase slowly as needed.
- Avoid adding drugs to treat side effects.
- Avoid using multiple medications from the same drug classifcation.
- Closely monitor medication changes for mental status alterations.

Chapter 5 discusses drug therapy for the elderly in detail.

To prevent delirium caused by hypoxia, supplemental oxygen should be administered. To minimize relocation trauma, such as would occur on admission to a hospital, the staff needs to consistently reorient the resident and provide emotional support as well as information. When possible, the resident should be managed in the nursing home.

Interventions for Residents with Delirium

When the nurse or other health care professional assesses sudden cognitive and emotional and/or behavioral changes in an elderly individual, delirium should be suspected. Determining the cause can be difficult, because more than one causative factor may contribute to this health problem. If a cause can be identified, it should be treated or removed if possible.

To help residents become or remain oriented, a structured environment that is safe and secure is essential. Resident participation in activities assists in keeping the residents alert. The activity program in a nursing home is coordinated by an activity therapist and includes both physical and mental activities. Further discussion about specific therapeutic activities is found in this chapter under "Dementia."

The most difficult aspect of delirium to manage is the behavioral component. The nurse and other staff need to continually orient the resident to reality and reassure the resident. Many individuals experience hallucinations, delusions, paranoia, and other psychotic symptoms that make them increasingly anxious and fearful. Specific interventions for these psychotic behaviors are described in this chapter under "Dementia."

DEPRESSION

Depression is the most common mental health problem among the elderly, especially those who live in nursing homes. An estimated 50 percent to 75 percent of residents in long term care have mild to moderate depression (Stanley & Beare, 1995). More accurate statistics are not available because most depressed residents are either misdiagnosed as having dementia or are not diagnosed at all.

Unfortunately, the negative consequences of depression can include a decreased quality of life, shortened life expectancy, or even suicide. The positive aspect of depression is that it is the most treatable mental health problem among the elderly.

Prevention of Depression

One of the best ways to prevent depression in a nursing home setting is to identify the groups most at risk. The highest incidence of depression among the elderly is found in Caucasian men between 75 and 85 years of age. They characteristically try to hide their illness and, in some cases, seek ways to commit suicide.

Other at-risk groups include residents with strokes or other physically disabling conditions and young adults with chronic, debilitating conditions, such as spinal cord injury or multiple sclerosis. The depression associated with stroke may be caused by a pathophysiologic change (organic cause) or may be a coping response to having a stroke (reactionary cause). Certain drugs can also cause a secondary depression. Examples include antihypertensive, cardiovascular, antiparkinsonian, and hypoglycemic agents, as well as alcohol and corticosteroids (Buckwalter & Babich, 1990).

After identifying residents at risk for depression, the nurse plans specific strategies to help prevent the illness. These interventions include displaying a caring attitude, and providing physical and social activities that make residents feel wanted and valued. Avoiding medications with known tendencies to cause depression is an important part of the care plan as well.

Assessment of Residents with Depression

Clinical depression is *not* the same as "having a bad day" or being temporarily sad. Depression is a mental health problem that must be properly diagnosed and treated. In the community, at least half of all depressed individuals are not identified as depressed by physicians (Sturm & Wells, 1995). Most depressed nursing home residents are initially identified by the nursing staff or family members rather than the physician, who is with residents for a limited period of time.

Residents with depression typically have poor self-esteem, display a loss of energy and interest in activities, and are in a persistently bad mood. They may be preoccupied with "being a burden" to the staff or family. In addition to these manifestations, depressed residents usually have a poor appetite, sleep disturbances, poor concentration, and lack of affect. Some residents become easily agitated or experience hallucinations. These characteristics contribute to the misdiagnosis of dementia (see discussion of dementia later in this chapter).

Although a number of rating scales to assess depression are available, the staff nurse in a nursing home setting may not have the opportunity to use them. Instead, the nurse needs to report significant manifestations to the health care provider for referral and treatment as soon as possible.

Interventions for Residents with Depression

Most physicians refer the resident suspected of having depression to a consulting psychiatrist or psychologist for a complete mental health evaluation. Once a diagnosis of depression is confirmed, individual treatment varies depending on the severity of the depression and other variables such as general health and age. Each treatment modality has advantages and disadvantages for the resident.

Psychotherapy or counseling is the least invasive treatment and may be useful for residents with mild to moderate depression. The clinical practice guidelines from the AHCPR state that psychotherapy usually requires at least 6 to 8 weeks to begin reducing symtoms associated with depression (Depression Guideline Panel, 1993). In addition, psychotherapy is very time-consuming and may be expensive.

For nursing home residents, drug therapy is commonly used to treat depression, with or without supplemental psychotherapy. Medications are easy to administer, take 4 to 6 weeks to work, and may be effective for mild, moderate, and severe depression. However, the adverse effects associated with these medications can be devastating, especially to elderly residents. Table 4–5 lists some of the commonly used agents and their adverse effects.

An alternative to drug therapy is electroconvulsive therapy (ECT)— the use of an electric shock to produce convulsions and loss of consciousness. The treatment reduces manifestations related to depression and is especially useful for individuals with severe depression; however, it is costly and has side effects such as short-term memory loss. Another disadvantage is that the resident may have other medical conditions that prohibit the use of ECT as a treatment (Depression Guideline Panel, 1993).

Table 4–5. **Adverse Effects of Medications Commonly Used to Treat Depression in the Elderly**

Medication	Adverse Effects (by Subgroup)
Tricyclic Antidepressants* Amitriptyline (Elavil, Endep) Clomipramine (Anafranil) Desipramine (Norpramin) Doxepin (Sinequan, Adapin) Imipramine (Tofranil) Nortriptyline (Pamelor) Protriptyline (Vivactil) Trimipramine (Surmontil)	Cardiac dysrhythmias, orthostatic hypotension, weight gain, drowsiness, anticholinergic effects (dry mouth, constipation, urinary retention, visual disturbances) (amitriptyline has the most anticholinergic effects of any in the group)
Heterocyclic Antidepressants† Amoxapine (Asendin) Bupropion (Wellbutrin) Maprotiline (Ludiomil) Trazadone (Desyrel)	Drowsiness (Maprotiline has the longest half-life of any in the group)
Selective Serotonin Reuptake Inhibitors (SSRIs)† Fluoxetine (Prozac) Paroxetine (Paxil) Sertraline (Zoloft)	Insomnia, agitation, gastrointestinal distress, weight loss (fluoxetine has the longest half-life on any in the group)
Monoamine Oxidase Inhibitors (MAOIs) Isocarboxazid (Maplan) Phenelzine (Nardil) Tranylcypromine (Parnate)	Weight gain, insomnia, agitation Hypertensive crisis (avoid food containing Tyromine)

*Do not give with antidysrhythmics or MAOIs.
†Do not give with MAOIs.
Data from *Depression in Primary Care: Volume 2. Treatment of Major Depression. Clinical Practice Guideline. Number 5.*

When treatment for the acute phase of the illness is complete, continuation and maintenance treatment may be necessary. Too often, though, a resident in a nursing home is placed on an antidepressant and the possibility of discontinuing the drug is never evaluated, even after symptoms of depression have diminished. The nurse can be an important advocate for the resident by keeping the physician informed of the resident's progress.

DEMENTIA

Unlike delirium and depression, dementia is a chronic, progressive impairment of cognitive function that may be accompanied by behavioral and emotional manifestations. It is typically not reversible and cannot be prevented. Dementia is also seen in some residents with acquired immunodeficiency syndrome (AIDS).

Dementia is a more current term than chronic brain syndrome (CBS) and organic brain syndrome (OBS). It is *not* a normal part of the aging process, but it does tend to occur primarily among the elderly. More than half of all nursing home residents have dementia; some facilities have specialty units where all of the residents have some type of dementia. Dementia can actually be considered as a symptom of many diseases, the most common of which is Alzheimer's disease.

Alzheimer's Disease

Alzheimer's disease accounts for more than half of all dementias among the elderly population and is the fourth leading cause of death in that population. When occurring among inidividuals over 65 years old, it is sometimes referred to as senile dementia, Alzheimer's type (SDAT). However, the term "senile" may suggest that when people get older they become cognitively impaired. Alzheimer's disease (AD) also affects a small percentage of individuals in their 40s and 50s. In this population it is referred to as presenile dementia, Alzheimer's type.

Although little is known about its exact cause, research has shown that the disease can run in families, a finding that suggests there may be a genetic or familial tendency in some cases. A gene that is thought to cause the most severe form of the disease has recently been identified. The older a person becomes, the greater are the chances of developing Alzheimer's disease. Nongenetic causes, such as viruses or aluminum, remain controversial.

The current estimate by the Alzheimer's Association is that more than 4 million people are affected by the disease. In the past, AD has been difficult to diagnose and may not have been confirmed until autopsy. The brain of a person with AD shows the characteristic plaques and neurofibrillary tangles. Today, diagnosis is easier because technological advances have provided tests, such as positron emission tomography (PET), that can support the diagnosis.

Although a number of staging schemes for AD are found in the literature, most experts stage the disease as early, middle, and late (Table 4–6). In the *early* stage of AD, the client experiences forgetfulness, especially short-term or recent memory loss. The individual can accurately describe an event that happened 30 years ago but cannot remember what he or she had for breakfast. At this stage, the individual is usually aware of the problem and may either deny it, fear it, or try to cover it up. Complex calculations, such as balancing a checkbook or keeping a golf score, become difficult. Judgment may also be impaired: for example, the person may forget to turn off the stove before going out. AD is very difficult to diagnose in this early stage.

As the disease progresses to the *middle* stage, personality changes increase. The usually calm, passive individual, for example, may become moody, irritable, or agitated. Problems with speech and language also

Table 4–6. **Causes of Confusion in the Elderly**

Neurologic Causes
  Vascular insufficiency
  Infections
  Trauma
  Tumors
  Normal pressure hydrocephalus

Cardiovascular Causes
  Myocardial infarction
  Dysrhythmias
  Congestive heart failure
  Cardiogenic shock
  Endocarditis

Pulmonary Causes
  Infection
  Pneumonia
  Hypoventilation

Metabolic Causes
  Electrolyte imbalance
  Acidosis/alkalosis
  Hypoglycemia/hyperglycemia
  Acute and chronic renal failure
  Fluid volume deficit
  Hepatic failure
  Porphyria

Drug Intoxication
  Misuse of prescribed medications
  Side effects of medications
  Incorrect use of over-the-counter medications
  Ingestion of heavy metals

Nutritional Deficiencies
  B vitamins
  Vitamin C
  Hypoproteinemia

Environmental Causes
  Hypothermia/hyperthermia
  Unfamiliar environment
  Sensory deprivation/overload

Psychologic Causes
  Depression
  Anxiety
  Pain
  Fatigue
  Grief
  Paranoia

begin to appear, especially aphasia (inability to speak) and anomia (inability to name objects). Emotional or behavioral manifestations, including hallucinations (imaginary visual, auditory, or olfactory perceptions) and delusions (false beliefs), can occur during the middle stage. Judgment is grossly impaired, and the individual begins to have difficulty with activities of daily living (ADLs). He or she may dress with three shirts and unmatched shoes. Attention to hygiene is lost and the individual is very confused. Symptoms worsen when the person is overstimulated.

During the *late* stage (terminal) of the illness, the person with AD experiences decreased mobility; incontinence of bowel and bladder; further impairment of memory, speech, and language; and emotional and/or behavioral responses, such as screaming or hallucinations. Convulsions may also occur among people in the middle and late stages of AD. Victims of AD die from complications of immobility, such as sepsis or pneumonia.

Other Types of Dementia

The second most common type of dementia is multi-infarct dementia. Unlike Alzheimer's disease, multi-infarct dementia is caused by a pathologic vascular problem. The individual, most often a middle-aged man, experiences multiple small strokes that impair cognitive ability.

Dementia may also be associated with chronic diseases such as Parkinson's disease, a common problem among the elderly, and Huntington's disease, a rare genetic disorder affecting younger adults. Regardless of the type of dementia, many of the behaviors and emotional responses of the resident are similar.

Assessment of Residents with Dementia

Dementia is usually not diagnosed in its earliest stages because manifestations begin slowly and may be subtle. The Alzheimer's Association has published the "Ten Warning Signs of AD," which are listed in Table 4–7. Several screening assessment tools are available for nurses, physicians, and

Table 4–7. **Ten Warning Signs of Alzheimer's Disease**

1. Recent memory loss affects job skills
2. Difficulty performing familiar tasks
3. Problems with language
4. Disorientation of time and place
5. Poor or decreased judgment
6. Misplacing things
7. Changes in mood or behavior
8. Changes in personality
9. Loss of initiative
10. Change in sleep pattern

other health care professionals. One of the most widely used is Folstein's Mini Mental-State Examination (MMSE), although other tools are also used. The MMSE (shown in Fig. 4–3) assesses mental status and has a maximum score of 30. A declining score is indicative of cognitive impairment.

Although easy to administer, the MMSE has the disadvantage of requiring that the resident have reasonable visual acuity and be able to read and write. A test that eliminates the need to read but offers less information on the severity of the cognitive impairment is the set test. In the set test, the nurse asks the resident to identify 10 items of a given set, such as 10 flowers, 10 vegetables, and so forth. Of course, the set selected by the examiner must be one that the individual would be familiar with. A demented resident is typically unable to state 10 items from a single set.

These assessment tools can help distinguish between depression and dementia. A depressed resident should be able to score better on the

Client _____ Examiner _____ Date _____

Maximum Score	Score	
		Orientation
5	( )	What is the (year) (season) (date) (day) (month)?
5	( )	Where are we (state) (country) (town) (hospital) (floor)?
		Registration
3	( )	Name 3 objects: 1 second to say each. Then ask the client all 3 after you have said them. Give 1 point for each correct answer. Then repeat them until he/she learns all 3. Count trials and record.
		Trials _____
		Attention and Calculation
5	( )	Serial 7's. 1 point for each correct answer. Stop after 5 answers. Alternatively spell "world" backward.
		Recall
3	( )	Ask for the 3 objects repeated above. Give 1 point for each correct answer.
		Language
2	( )	Name a pencil and watch. (2 points)
1	( )	Repeat the following "No ifs, ands, or buts." (1 point)
3	( )	Follow a 3-stage command: "Take a paper in your hand, fold it in half, and put it on the floor." (3 points)
1	( )	Read and obey the following: CLOSE YOUR EYES. (1 point)
1	( )	Write a sentence. (1 point)
1	( )	Copy design. (1 point)
_____		Total Score

Figure 4–3. The Mini Mental-State Examination used to assess cognitive function.

MMSE and set test than a resident with dementia. Some demented individuals also experience depression. Many nursing homes encourage or require the use of the MMSE or a similar tool to identify dementia in previously undiagnosed residents or to determine the progress of the disease.

A complete medical workup is usually scheduled for a person suspected of having dementia. In addition to a history and physical examination, a number of tests may be ordered, such as a computed tomography (CT) scan or the more sophisticated PET scan or SPECT (single positron emission computed tomography) scan if these are available. These scans show the size of the brain (which decreases about 5 percent with age, but is decreased by 8 percent to 10 percent in persons with Alzheimer's disease). The PET and SPECT scans determine neuronal activity in the brain.

Interventions for Residents with Dementia

Individuals with early stage dementia usually reside in the community and are supervised by family or other caregiver support system, such as adult day care. As the disease progresses, though, behaviors such as hallucinations, wandering, or sleep-wake disturbance may encourage the family to seek nursing home placement, often in a dementia unit. Physical problems such as decreased ability to perform ADLs and incontinence may also initiate placement in a long term care facility.

Care planning for the resident must be individualized, because all residents with dementia do not manifest the same behaviors. Some residents are confused but do not have any associated atypical behaviors. Others have multiple problems which pose a challenge to nursing staff.

The primary interventions for residents with dementia are environmental restructuring, validation therapy, avoidance of triggers that aggravate behaviors, and managing difficult behaviors.

Ripich, Wykle, and Niles (1995) advocate a FOCUSED approach to communication with people experiencing dementia:

F = Face-to-face interaction
O = Orientation (if feasible)
C = Continuity of care and staff
U = Unsticking (helping residents find the words they want to use)
S = Structure
E = Exchange (interaction)
D = Direct approach

Environmental Restructuring

The environment must be secure, structured, and calm because the demented resident is typically fearful and anxious. The resident should be kept away from the nurses' station or other high-traffic areas. The nursing home staff must be educated regarding the need to avoid shouting or other loud noises. All staff must take responsibility for the resident's safety and redirect the individual as needed. A hug or gentle touch can provide a sense of security and caring.

Structure and consistency in the environment is crucial. For example, a daily routine for each resident is established and maintained. In the environment, calming blues and greens are better than reds and oranges.

Demented residents benefit from consistent staff who provide care. In a nursing home setting, the nurse should consider this need when making staff assignments.

Structured therapeutic activities are important to provide distraction, mild stimulation, enjoyment, and social interaction. For example, musical activities and art can be used for any stage of dementia. For residents who have do not have speech and language problems, making word substitutions in familiar songs is an appropriate activity. For middle stage dementia, exercising or dancing to music can be fun. For severely demented residents who have decreased mobility, listening to their favorite music can be very therapeutic.

Validation Therapy

One of the most important interventions for any resident with a cognitive impairment is to communicate with the individual, even if he or she is severely demented. For people with early dementia in whom periods of lucidity are common, orientation to reality, as discussed in this chapter under "Delirium," may be useful. However, for residents with middle or late stage dementia, reality orientation is not effective and can actually increase agitation or other emotional responses.

As described by Naomi Feil (1993), validation therapy is the most appropriate way to communicate with individuals who are demented. It involves respect for the person's feelings and beliefs, and confirming them rather than disputing them. For example, a resident who insists that he has not been given his breakfast (although he just ate all of it) will become agitated if he is told that he cannot have any food because he has just eaten. Using validation therapy, the staff shows concern and acknowledges that the resident feels he is hungry. The resident may be offered more food, preferably food that he chooses.

If the resident has a visual hallucination in which he thinks there are bugs on the ceiling, the nurse acknowledges the bugs and may need to find a way to eliminate them. If the nurse insists that the bugs are not present, the resident will be afraid and not trust the nurse.

Avoiding Behavior Triggers

Many of the behavioral or emotional responses experienced by residents with dementia are aggravated or triggered by certain factors. A nursing intervention, then, is to identify the trigger for the resident and avoid it, if possible, in the future. If the trigger cannot be avoided, it should be treated or removed as quickly as possible.

Examples of factors that can worsen or cause these responses include acute illnesses, such as pneumonia, hypoglycemia, or myocardial infarction. These problems decrease oxygen supply to the brain or cause toxins to affect the brain. Environmental and/or sensory factors—such as pain, drugs (especially chemical restraints), decreased visual or hearing acuity, and relocation—can also initiate or increase problem behaviors. Other factors include lack of sleep and use of physical restraints.

In many cases, the resident is unable to communicate what the trigger is to the nurse. The nurse must anticipate possible factors contributing to the behavior and act accordingly. For example, if the resident has severe arthritis, providing a drug for pain relief may resolve the problem behavior.

Managing Difficult Behaviors

Behavioral problems vary among residents with dementia. Common problems, though, include wandering, screaming, wanting to "go home," agitation, sleep disturbances, and problems with performing activities of daily living. The presence of staff, family, or loved ones may help to calm the resident who is manifesting difficult behaviors, such as severe agitation. Woods and Ashley (1995) found that audiotapes of loved ones helped comfort the resident and manage problem behaviors. This simulated presence therapy was more effective than the staff's presence in calming the residents.

Table 4–8 lists several common problem behaviors and strategies for managing them.

Use of Physical and Chemical Restraints

In the past, restraints were used as a common intervention for confused residents to prevent falls. Restraints are any physical device or chemical agent that prevents the resident from moving at will. Between one-third and two-thirds of all nursing home residents in the United States were restrained in 1990. Fewer than 4 percent of residents were restrained in European countries such as England, Sweden, and Denmark (Powell, 1993).

As a result of these alarming statistics, the federal Omnibus Budget Reconciliation Act (OBRA) of 1987 mandated that residents in nursing homes have the right to be free of both physical and chemical restraints (psychotropic drugs). Research showed that although nursing staff thought they were protecting residents through the use of physical restraints, they were causing serious injuries, including death. A number of choking deaths from vest restraints, falls, fractures, and bruises prompted federal legislation that went into effect in October 1990.

Table 4–8. **Management of Common Problem Behaviors Associated with Dementia**

Problem Behavior	Key Interventions
Angry, agitated behavior or screaming	Reduce stimulation in the environment, such as excessive noise, clutter, or people. Keep a consistent daily routine; avoid changes. Remove the resident from stressful situations. Distract the resident with a favorite food or activity. Try music or massage to calm the resident. Use gentle touch. Check for physical cause of behavior, such as pain.
Wandering	Provide opportunities for exercise, singing, or dancing. Provide secured indoor and outdoor areas for wandering. Decrease environmental stimulation. Reinforce location of public areas and bathroom using bright labels or colors. Toilet the resident every 2 hours, or more often if needed. Place a plastic strip across the doors to prevent wandering outside, or use stop sign or NO! sign on door. Distract with food or activity. Do not restrain the resident, as restraint increases stress and abuses resident's rights.
Hallucinations and/or paranoia	Have vision or glasses checked. Have hearing or hearing aid checked. Assess for physical cause of behavior. Increase lighting. Avoid abstract artwork and wallpaper. Use familiar or favorite distractions. Communicate with the resident in a reassuring tone of voice. Use gentle touch. Do not disagree or argue with the resident.

Physical Restraints

Since 1990, a tremendous educational effort regarding restraints has taken place throughout the nursing home industry. Facilities and vendors have sought to develop less restrictive devices that could ensure safety while maintaining the resident's rights. Although a handful of nursing homes are "restraint free," most are "restraint appropriate." This term means that restraints are used only as a last resort and then the least restrictive device is used.

The best intervention, of course, is to use no restraints, including bedrails. Facilities that have accomplished this goal use alternatives such as letting residents sleep on mattresses on the floor; using reclining chairs, wedges, and pillows; and placing brightly colored tape or stop signs at doors to prevent wanderers from leaving the building. Door alarms alert the staff to opening doors.

Some facilities, however, have a large percentage of residents with severe dementia or other cognitive impairment. For these residents, using the least restrictive devices like "Lap Buddies" provides a safe yet gentle reminder to get out of a chair with assistance. Merry Walkers (walkers that enclose the resident and allow them to sit as needed) and safety belts can be used for ambulatory residents. Toileting patients at 1- to 2-hour intervals also decreases the need to get out of bed or a chair without help. In addition, it is necessary to place the call light close by the resident at all times and to give frequent reminders about using it for assistance.

Chemical Restraints

Chemical restraints (psychotropic drugs) cause equally negative outcomes. Most psychotropic drugs used to calm confused residents have a long list of adverse effects, including hallucinations, hypotension, constipation, dry mouth, decreased physical activity, increased confusion, sedation, and tardive dyskinesia. The latter is an irreversible syndrome of automatic, rhythmic movements that cannot be controlled by the individual (e.g., pill-rolling motion with the fingers, lip smacking).

Residents who are placed on psychotropics must have a baseline assessment and be monitored closely for adverse effects, such as tardive dyskinesia. An assessment tool (such as the abnormal involuntary movement scale [AIMS] test) is usually completed every 6 months to document any changes. The offending drug should be discontinued if adverse effects occur.

Like physical restraints, chemical restraints may need to be administered on a short-term basis for certain residents as a last resort. Most of the drugs listed in Table 4–9 are used to control difficult behaviors such as severe agitation, hallucinations, and delusions. They do not treat the dementia, but rather attempt to control the behaviors associated with dementia or delirium.

Several new drugs are being used to improve memory and function of residents with Alzheimer's disease. These medications enhance the action of acetycholine in the brain to improve neuronal activity.

Malnutrition

A major concern regarding residents in nursing homes is nutritional status. Obesity is more likely to occur in younger residents who are wheel-

Table 4–9. **Drugs Commonly Used as Chemical Restraints**

Low Potency (high sedation, high anticholinergic effects)
Chlorpromazine (Thorazine)
Thioridazine (Mellaril)
Chlorprothixene (Tractan)
Mesoridazine (Serentil)

Medium Potency (medium sedation, medium anticholinergic effects)
Triflupromazine (Vesprin)
Acetophenazine (Tindal)
Loxapine (Loxitane)
Molindone (Moban)

High Potency (low sedation, low anticholinergic effects)
Trifluoperazine (Stelazine)
Thiothixene (Navane)
Fluphenazine (Prolixin)
Haloperidol (Haldol)
Pimozide (Orap)

chair bound or otherwise immobilized. Decreased mobility combined with overeating can easily cause weight gain. Excess weight can be a hinderance when the resident transfers from bed to chair or vice versa. Although some residents may be obese, the most common nutrition problem in a nursing home setting is typically undernutrition or malnutrition, especially among the elderly population. Undernutrition is suspected if the resident loses more than 5 pounds in a month or has a 10 percent weight loss over 6 months. Fluid loss from diuresis can also result in marked weight loss, and laboratory assessment helps to identify the cause of the weight change.

Many severely ill elderly residents are at risk for protein-calorie malnutrition (PCM), also called protein-energy malnutrition, a severe form of undernutrition. In this condition, the resident has a deficiency of both protein and calories. The body breaks down tissues (protein catabolism), causing a negative nitrogen balance, weight loss, weakness, and skeletal muscle wasting. Weight loss and malnutrition in the elderly contribute to medical complications and death among the elderly in any health care setting (American Society of Parenteral and Enteral Nutrition [ASPEN], 1993). Some of the common complications include anemia, edema, poor wound healing, increased infection rate, decreased energy, intolerance to cold, alopecia (hair loss), and in severe cases, cachexia—a generalized wasting of body tissues.

Malnutrition is actually more common in hospitalized individuals than among nursing home residents. Nursing homes staff must follow strict federal and state regulations regarding nutritional requirements and weight monitoring. Hospitals, on the other hand, may not focus on nutrition as a top priority, which may explain the high incidence of PCM in these settings. As many as 50 percent of hospitalized individuals have moderate malnutrition and 5 percent to 10 percent have severe malnutrition (ASPEN, 1993).

PREVENTION OF MALNUTRITION

As discussed for the previous health problems, one of the best ways to prevent difficulties is to first identify the most at-risk individuals. The elderly with chronic diseases, problems with digestion or intestinal absorption, difficulties in swallowing or chewing, and anorexia are the residents most likely to develop malnutrition.

In taking a nutritional history, the nurse asks about complaints of heartburn or nausea with eating. Dental health also needs to be assessed. Many of today's elderly are edentulous (without natural teeth) because they did not have access to preventive dental care when they were younger. Tooth loss is *not* a normal physiologic change associated with aging.

If the resident has dentures or partial plates, he or she needs an evaluation of their fit. When people lose weight, dentures become loose, causing discomfort for the resident. If needed, the resident should be seen by a dentist for new dentures or care for diseased teeth or gums.

ASSESSMENT OF RESIDENTS WITH MALNUTRITION

A nutritional assessment consists of a complete physical assessment, food intake evaluation, weight monitoring, and laboratory assessment. In addition to noting changes in physical condition that may indicate complications as described above, the nursing staff monitor and record the percentage of meals that each resident consumes each day. For a more detailed intake record, the dietitian may request that the staff record all food and liquid portions consumed over a consecutive 3- to 7-day period.

Weight and Height

Weights may be taken daily, weekly, or monthly, depending on the resident's status. If the difference between weekly or monthly weights is 5 pounds or more, the resident should be reweighed. If weight loss occurs, the next step is to determine whether the weight change was the result of a fluid loss rather than actual loss in body mass. Residents with edema from congestive heart failure or other fluid retention disorders are often placed on diuretics and should lose weight as urinary output increases. The best indicator of fluid gain or loss is weight change. Chapter 6 discusses fluid imbalances in detail.

The resident's weight is also compared to ideal body weight (IBW) or usual body weight (UBW). Ideal body weights come from a predetermined table, such as the Metropolitian Life Height and Weight Table. Some individuals, however, have never had a weight as high as IBW in their lives and are not likely to reach that goal in a nursing home. In these cases, UBW may be a more realistic goal.

In addition to weight, some dietitians use body mass index (BMI) for evaluating nutritional status. This measure does not depend on body frame and estimates total fat stores within the body by the relationship of weight and height. One formula for calculating BMI is:

$$BMI = \frac{weight^2 \ (kg^2)}{height^2 \ (m^2)}$$

A BMI between 20 and 25 is desirable (Mahan & Arlin, 1992).

One of the problems with measuring the height of residents in a nursing home is that many individuals are unable to stand to have their height assessed. Therefore, other measures or estimates of height are needed. For the resident who can lie supine and is not contracted, using a tape measure to assess height while the resident is in bed is the best alternative. If the resident is contracted, however, this method does not work. Several devices, including a knee caliper, can be utilized to estimate height. By measuring the length of the lower leg with a knee caliper and using a scale or formula, the resident's height can be fairly accurately estimated. The dietitian can recommend the best device to purchase for the facility. An accurate height measurement is extremely important in determining a goal for the resident's weight or for calculating the BMI.

Skin Fold Measurements

The dietitian may also estimate body fat by performing a series of skin fold measurements. The triceps and subscapular skin folds are most frequently used, and the measurements are compared to predetermined standards. In most nursing homes, though, the dietitian does not usually have the time to use this particular evaluation method for every resident. Laboratory assessment may be more helpful in monitoring nutritional state.

Laboratory Tests

Routine laboratory tests can provide additional or supporting information about a resident's nutritional status. For example, a low hemoglobin and hematocrit is indicative of anemia. Although there are a number of reasons for anemia, a malnourished resident typically has anemia, as well as a decreased serum iron level.

Individuals experiencing malnutrition also have a depressed immune system, making them susceptible to infections. The white blood cell count may diminish, especially the lymphocyte component, which is responsible for making antibodies.

Malnutrition markedly affects serum protein levels. Serum albumin reflects the body's protein status but is not an early indicator that the resident is undernourished. By the time the serum albumin drops, the resident has been in a malnourished state for several weeks or longer. A low albumin also contributes to a shift of body fluid out of the intravascular space (bloodstream) and into the interstitial tissues. The resulting peripheral edema may mask the muscle wasting that is typical of severe malnutrition.

Earlier indications of decreased nutritional status are reflected in the serum transferrin and thyroxine-binding prealbumin (PAB) values. Serum transferrin is an iron-transport protein and can either be measured directly or estimated by using a formula. Thyroxine PAB is the best indicator because it is affected in just a few days after a malnourished state begins. However, this test is expensive and is not available in all laboratories (Viall, 1995).

Serum cholesterol has received a significant amount of attention in relationship to heart disease. An increased level is one of many risk factors for cardiovascular health problems. However, a low cholesterol level can be problematic as well, especially for an elderly person. Cholesterol levels decrease in a number of chronic diseases, including malabsorption, liver disesae, terminal cancer, malnutrition, and sepsis. The individual with a low cholesterol level has decreased healing ability. Table 4–10 summarizes the laboratory findings for residents with malnutrition.

INTERVENTIONS FOR RESIDENTS WITH MALNUTRITION

For the resident with malnutrition, the dietitian, in collaboration with the health care team, establishes goals for weight and laboratory values. Then, an individualized plan to meet the goals is developed.

If the resident is able to ingest food orally, the diet usually includes foods high in protein and calories in small, frequent feedings. If necessary,

Table 4–10. **Common Laboratory Findings in Residents with Malnutrition**

Serum Laboratory Test	Finding
Hemoglobin and hematocrit	Decreased
White blood cell count (especially lymphocytes)	Decreased
Total protein	Decreased
Albumin	Decreased
Transferrin	Decreased (early)
Thyroxine prealbumin (PAB)	Decreased (early)
Cholesterol	Decreased

between-meal snacks, such as cheese and crackers, instant breakfast drinks, or milkshakes, can be added to meet daily requirements.

Partial Enteral Nutrition

Some residents receive additional enteral products, such as Ensure or Ensure Plus, to supplement the prescribed diet. These solutions are high in protein, calories, and other nutrients, providing 1 to 2 calories/mL. Most supplements are now available in various flavors, such as vanilla, strawberry, and chocolate. Commercial puddings with the same nutritional value or candy bars are sometimes better accepted by the resident.

Other options may be needed for residents with special health problems. For example, Glucerna is a product designed especially for residents with diabetes mellitus. Special products are also available for residents in renal failure or for those with chronic pulmonary disease. For residents who are on fluid restriction or cannot tolerate additional fluid, powdered modular supplements may be given. Examples of these products are ProPac or ProMod for protein supplementation and Polycose for carbohydrate supplementation. Depending on need, several scoops of the powder are mixed in any fluid that the resident will drink.

Total Enteral Nutrition

If the resident is unable to meet the nutritional goals through oral intake, total enteral nutrition (TEN) through a feeding tube may be required. Other candidates for TEN include residents who have permanent neuromuscular impairment and cannot swallow, and those in a coma, persistent vegetative state, or terminal stage of illness.

Ethical Considerations

The ethical dilemma surrounding the use of feeding tubes is growing as people are living longer and health care costs soar. A particularly difficult choice is presented when recovery is unlikely. In this case, is tube feeding a death-delaying rather than a life-prolonging treatment?

Some experts argue that nutrition is a basic need that must be met. Others believe that tube feeding is a medical procedure that can be withheld if there is no possible medical benefit. Many nurses are uncomfortable about withholding food and water but have seen the multiple medical complications that can lead to death from tube feeding (Bosek & Savage, 1995). The dilemma is less troublesome if the resident has an advance directive (power of attorney for health care) that specifies what his or her wishes are in the event that the resident is not able to verbalize those wishes when necessary. Chapter 15 discusses advance directives in detail.

Feeding Tubes

Total enteral nutrition, also referred to as "tube feeding," can be administered through a variety of tubes. For short-term use, nasogastric (NG) tubes are often appropriate. As the name implies, the tube is passed through the nares and into the stomach. An improved type of nasoenteral tube that can be used for feeding is the nasoduodenal (ND) tube. Compared to NG tubes, these tubes are typically of smaller bore (diameter), are softer and more pliable, and descend into the duodenum with the help of a small weight at the end of the tube. Both the NG and ND tubes can be inserted by nurses.

To help reduce the risk of aspiration of contents into the lungs, a gastrostomy tube (G-tube) is often the alternative for a resident on long-term tube feeding. The G-tube can be inserted surgically through a small incision, laparoscopically, or percutaneously through an endoscope. Percutaneous endoscopic gastrostomy (PEG) tubes are becoming very popular because they do not require a surgical incision. The initial gastrostomy tube is placed by the physician. If the resident has a Foley catheter used as a G-tube, the nurse may replace the tube or change the tube if it becomes dislodged. Otherwise, replacements of G-tubes must be performed by the health care provider.

Although the possibility of aspiration is minimized by using a G-tube, the risk of infection is higher when a surgical incision is required. For residents who do not have a stomach or have had a large portion of the stomach removed, a jejunostomy tube (J-tube) can be inserted into the jejunum in the same manner as the G-tube. J-tubes are not commonly used but provide an alternative if residents need them.

After any feeding tube is initially inserted, its placement must be verified by x-ray. During the course of nutritional therapy, the nurse must check tube placement periodically, usually before any feeding or medication is administered, or every 4 hours when the resident receives continuous feeding. Placement may be checked by aspirating gastric contents using a piston syringe. If no contents are aspirated, moving the resident to a side-lying position may facilitate the process.

Recent nursing research has demonstrated that the auscultatory method commonly used to assess placement is not reliable for residents with small bore tubes. Using this method, the nurse injects about 30 mL of air into the tube while listening over the cardia of the stomach with a stethoscope for a swooshing sound. For small bore tubes, the sound may be heard even if the tube is dislodged into the lungs. Therefore, it has been recommended that the stomach aspirate be tested for pH as a more reliable method for checking tube placement. If the placement is correct, the pH will be low because the gastric contents contain acid. Duodenal contents are more alkaline (Fater, 1995).

An important additional nursing intervention for residents with G-tubes is to change the dressing around the tube and monitor the skin for signs of inflammation or infection. If severe redness or drainage is present, the physician should be notified.

Feeding Products

A number of commercially prepared products are available for total enteral nutrition. The choice of product depends on the resident's nutritional needs. Many formulas, such as Jevity and Osmolite, provide 1 calorie/mL of solution. More concentrated formulas like TwoCal HN provide 2 calories/mL and a higher protein content. The dietitian, in collaboration with the physician, determines the appropriate formula for each resident.

When the feeding begins, the formula may be diluted to help the resident's digestive tract adapt to the feeding. Additional water is also prescribed to help meet the resident's fluid needs. Unless the resident needs a fluid restriction, 30 mL/kg of body weight is usually recommended (Shelton & Ignatavicius, 1995).

Feeding Methods

Three methods for tube feeding are used—bolus, continuous, and cyclic (cycled). A requirement for all three methods is that the resident must be in a semi-Fowler or sitting position to help prevent aspiration before, during, and after each feeding.

The *bolus* feeding method is the oldest available method and is used less commonly in nursing home settings than the continuous or cyclic methods. The nurse checks for placement and residual gastric contents before giving the feeding. If a large amount of fluid is aspirated from the stomach (over 100 mL), the feeding may be delayed. The residual contents are returned to the stomach.

If the residual volume is less than 100 mL, the nurse administers the prescribed amount of formula and water at specified intervals, often every 4 hours. The solution can be given through a large syringe by gravity or via a mechanical pump or controller. Rapid administration should be avoided because it tends to cause discomfort and may cause diarrhea, a common complication of total enteral nutrition. After the feeding, additional water is given as ordered, usually 50 to 75 mL every 4 hours for hydration.

The *continuous* feeding method requires the use of a mechanical food pump to administer a prescribed hourly amount of formula. The formula is placed in a feeding administration bag and connected to an administration set designed to fit the pump. No more than a 24-hour supply of formula should be placed in the feeding bag. Some facilities use prefilled plastic containers that contain the prescribed formula. Each container must hang for less than 24 hours to prevent bacterial growth and possible contamination. The administration set must also be changed every 24 hours.

A resident on continuous feeding should be monitored carefully. Every 4 hours, the tube is typically checked for placement, the resident is checked for residual gastric contents, and the tube is flushed with water. If diarrhea occurs, the formula may need to be slowed, diluted, or changed. Some formulas are hyperosmolar, and the pulling of fluid from the intestines by these formula causes diarrhea.

The *cyclic* feeding method is similar to continuous feeding except that the infusion does not continue around the clock. Instead, a "down time" of 4 to 8 hours allows the digestive tract to rest and allows the staff the opportunity to provide personal care, treatments, and so forth while the feeding is interrupted. This method is very popular in most nursing homes. Table 4–11 lists typical physician's orders for a resident receiving cyclic tube feeding in a nursing home.

Complications Associated with Tube Feeding

The nurse monitors the resident for complications that can result from total enteral nutrition. Some problems are related to the tube while others are related to the formula.

The most common complication related to the *tube* is clogging from concentrated formula or medication. To prevent clogging, the nurse should use liquid medications rather than attempting to flush crushed pills through the tube (Table 4–12). Warm water is better than cold for flushing. If the tube becomes clogged, administering 30 mL of warm water in a piston syringe using gentle pressure often resolves the problem. Carbonated beverages should be used to unclog the tube only as a last resort. If the tube becomes clogged frequently, the formula or medications should be changed.

Aspiration pneumonia is another common tube complication, especially for residents with nasogastric or nasoduodenal tubes. Keeping the resident upright at an angle of at least 30 degrees and checking placement on a regular basis help to minimize the risk of pneumonia.

Table 4–11. **Information Included in Physician's Orders for Enteral Nutrition**

- Amount and type of formula; total calories for 24 hours
- Method of feeding administration (bolus, continuous, or cyclic)
- How often feeding is to be given (specify "down time" for cyclic feeding per 24 hours)
- Amount of water used for flushing and flushing interval
- Amount of additional water to be given and how often
- Frequency for residual checks; what to do if residual is present
- How often feeding administration set should be changed
- How often feeding tube is to be changed

Table 4–12. Tips for Administering Medications Through a Feeding Tube

- Check tube placement before each medication administration.
- If the resident receives continuous or cyclic feedings and needs a drug to be administered on an empty stomach, stop the feeding for at least 15 minutes before giving the drug and do not restart the feeding for 1 hour after administering the drug.
- Do not administer enteric-coated medications through a feeding tube and do not crush them.
- Do not crush slow-release drugs; instead, open the capsule and flush its contents through a large-bore tube. Do not give these drugs through a small-bore tube.
- When giving nifedipine (Procardia), make a small hole in the capsule with a needle and squeeze the contents down the tube.
- Do not administer sublingual medications, such as nitroglycerin (Nitrostat), through the tube; they should be absorbed in the mouth.
- When giving an antacid, wait 30–60 minutes after giving cimetidine (Tagamet), tetracycline, or iron.
- Do not administer bulking agents (e.g., Metamucil) through a feeding tube.
- Flush the tube before and after *each* medication with 15–30 mL of water.
- Give one medication at a time and flush between each one.

In addition to diarrhea, fluid and electrolyte imbalances may result from the feeding *formula*. Weights should be monitored frequently and laboratory values for protein, electrolytes, and complete blood count should be obtained periodically to evaluate the effectiveness of the nutritional therapy.

Documentation for Tube Feeding

In addition to recording the amount of formula and water given, the amount of residual must be recorded on the intake and output record. Any medical complications or omissions of the feeding must also be documented, with the reason, if known. The nurse also records tube changes and notes weight and laboratory test changes. If the resident is able to comprehend, teaching about the tube feeding should be recorded in the medical record as well.

Parenteral Nutrition

The preferred route for nutrients is the gastrointestinal (GI) tract. However, if the resident is unable to use the GI tract for nutrition, parenteral nutrition is necessary. Conventional solutions used for maintenance intravenous (IV) therapy typically contain 5 percent to 10 percent dextrose, or 170 to 340 calories/L, respectively. Therefore, to adequately meet the body's nutritional needs, more concentrated solutions containing dextrose, amino acids (protein), fats, vitamins, and minerals are required. This method of meeting nutritional needs is called parenteral nutrition.

Nursing homes are increasingly admitting residents needing parenteral nutrition. Parenteral nutrition, also called hyperalimentation or "hyper," may be partial or total.

Partial Parenteral Nutrition

Partial parenteral nutrition (PPN) is usually administered to residents who are unable to fulfill their nutritional requirements by oral intake alone. It is delivered via a large peripheral vein through a cannula or catheter. Amino acid–dextrose solutions (usually 10%) and lipid (fat) emulsions (usually 10% to 20%) are given to provide PPN. Vitamins and minerals are added to this solution as needed for each resident.

A fairly new product for PPN is a mixture of amino acids, dextrose, and lipids, sometimes called a 3:1 solution, triple-mix solution, or total nutrient admixture (TNA) (Weinstein, 1993). TNA is prepared in a 3 liter bag and administered via an electronic infusion device. An in-line filter of at least 1.2 microns is needed to allow fat particles to pass (Viall, 1995). Another important consideration for lipid infusion is to determine whether the resident has an allergy to eggs or a history of fat embolism syndrome because in either case lipids are contraindicated.

Total Parenteral Nutrition

Total parenteral nutrition (TPN) is used for residents requiring extensive nutritional support for a specified but prolonged period of time. It is administered by central venous access device (VAD) because the solution used has much higher amino acid and dextrose concentrations than the PPN solution. These high concentrations result in a very hyperosmolar solution, with an osmolarity about 3 to 6 times greater than that of blood. Like PPN solutions, TPN solutions also contain essential vitamins and minerals needed by the body. The pharmacist is usually responsible for mixing the solutions used for both TPN and PPN. Insulin may be added to compensate for the high concentration of dextrose.

Complications of Parenteral Nutrition

The most common complication of parenteral nutrition is infection, especially in residents with central venous access devices, such as tunneled catheters or multi-lumen catheters (Fig. 4–4). The high concentrations of glucose and amino acids makes the exit site an ideal area for bacterial growth. Proper handwashing and strict sterile technique help decrease the chance of infection.

Complications related to the catheter may also occur, such as dislodgement or malpositioning, breakage, or occlusion. More commonly, though, metabolic complications resulting from the solutions are seen in elderly residents. Examples include hyper- or hypoglycemia, fluid overload, prerenal azotemia (elevated blood urea nitrogen [BUN] from the increased amino acids), and electrolyte imbalances. Table 4–13 lists nursing interventions that help prevent or detect complications of parenteral nutrition.

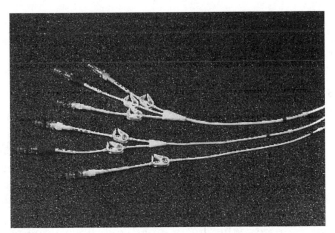

Figure 4-4. *Hickman peripherally inserted central catheters.* From *Medical-Surgical Nursing: A Nursing Process Approach* (p. 278), by D. D. Ignatavicius, M. L. Workman, and M. A. Mishler, 1995, Philadelphia: W. B. Saunders. Reprinted with permission.

Table 4–13. **Nursing Interventions Associated with Parenteral Nutrition Therapy**

- Carefully check each bag or bottle of solution for accuracy against the physician's order.
- Check the TPN solution for "cracking" (i.e., separation of the fluid into layers); do not use if cracked.
- Monitor the accuracy of the electronic infusion device by marking the solution container in hourly increments.
- If the solution is "behind," do not increase the rate to get it back on schedule.
- Check the IV puncture site carefully for signs of infection and placement.
- Start TPN slowly and taper it slowly to prevent major changes in serum glucose levels; a recommended flow rate is one-half of the prescribed rate for 1 hour before discontinuing.
- Weigh the patient every day early in the morning.
- Monitor laboratory values carefully, especially BUN, creatinine, electrolytes, and glucose, which are typically drawn daily for the first 3–7 days, then twice a week.
- Monitor liver enzmes every 3–4 days.
- Record the patient's intake and output carefully.
- Observe for signs and symptoms of complications, such as crackles in patients with congestive heart failure.
- Monitor blood glucose and vital signs every 4–6 hours or as specified by the agency or physician.
- Administer vitamin K as ordered for clotting because TPN solution does not contain vitamin K.
- Change the IV administration set according to agency policy, usually every 24–72 hours.
- If new TPN solution is not available, administer dextrose 10% until the next TPN container is ready.

From *Stroot's Fluids and Electrolytes: A Practical Approach* (p.219), by C. A. Lee, A. Barrett, and D. D. Ignatavicius, 1996, Philadelphia : F. A. Davis. Reprinted with permission.

Constipation

Constipation is a very common problem among elderly and immobilized residents. It may be defined as difficult or infrequent defecation, with uncomfortable passage of dry, hard stool.

FACTORS CONTRIBUTING TO CONSTIPATION

Decreased gastrointestinal motility and decreased physical mobility place the elderly resident at high risk for constipation. Other risk factors include improper diet, inadequate fluid intake, and drugs that cause constipation, such as anticholinergics, iron preparations, and antacids containing magnesium. In addition, some elderly residents have a history of laxative abuse due to the belief that they must have a daily bowel movement to be healthy. Prolonged use of laxatives causes the intestinal wall to lose muscle tone.

Younger residents who are immobilized, have impaired physical mobility, or are taking anticholinergics or codeine-containing drugs are also at a high risk for constipation. The presence of hemorrhoids increases the discomfort associated with the passage of hard stool.

Any resident who is constipated is at risk for intestinal obstruction, a severe, life-threatening complication. Constipation is also a risk factor for colon cancer.

PREVENTION OF CONSTIPATION

Aggressive prevention of constipation is essential for nursing home residents. Increased fluids (at least 1500 mL/day), dietary fiber, and exercise, to the extent possible, are provided for every resident, unless otherwise contraindicated for a medical condition. The dietitian, in collaboration with the nurse, plans the appropriate dietary intervention, which often includes prunes or prune juice (although this practice is currently controversial), bran, and fresh fruits and vegetables to provide high fiber in the diet. Some facilities use additional interventions such as high-fiber cookies or a mixture of applesauce, prune juice, and bran administered to residents on a daily basis. Recommended daily fiber intake is between 12 and 20 g (Brown & Everett, 1990). Warm liquids with meals may help stimulate elimination.

Additional prevention measures include establishing a bowel routine, usually every other day. Establishing such a routine is facilitated by toileting residents after meals, especially after breakfast. Providing privacy is particularly important. If possible, the resident should sit on a commode or sit upright on the bedpan, in a position in which gravity assists the passage of stool.

Pharmacologic intervention is usually used only for residents who have a history of constipation or are suffering from actual constipation, and when other measures have failed. It should not be used routinely as part of the prevention plan.

ASSESSMENT OF RESIDENTS WITH CONSTIPATION

In the nursing home setting, every resident's bowel movements are recorded so that problems can be detected early. The size and consistency of the stool should be recorded as well. For example, some residents may have small diarrheal-type stools, which can be indicative of an impaction. In an impaction, a mass of hard stool becomes lodged in the sigmoid colon or rectum. Stool then leaks around the impaction, which must be removed before it causes an intestinal obstruction. If the size and nature of the stools are recorded, the nurse is alerted to the need for a digital examination to confirm the presence of an impaction.

The resident with an impaction or obstruction also usually presents with a distended, uncomfortable abdomen. The nurse performs an abdominal assessment, being sure to listen to bowel sounds *before* palpating the abdomen. Bowel sounds may be decreased, indicating slowed peristalsis, or increased, indicating the bowel's attempt to push the stool past the area of impaction or obstruction. If the resident has an intestinal obstruction, bowel sounds may be absent, especially below the site of the obstruction. Table 4–14 lists the assessment findings associated with large-bowel and small-bowel obstructions.

INTERVENTIONS FOR RESIDENTS WITH CONSTIPATION

Management of constipation includes the preventive measures described earlier, as well as pharmacologic intervention. When possible, stool softeners, such as Colace, or gentle laxatives, such as Senekot, should be administered. Some residents, especially those with an impaction, require more aggressive interventions, such as laxatives, suppositories, and enemas.

Table 4–14. **Key Features of Small-Bowel and Large-Bowel Obstruction**

Small-Bowel Obstruction	Large-Bowel Obstruction
■ Abdominal discomfort/pain, possibly accompanied by visible peristaltic waves in upper and mid abdomen	■ Severe lower abdominal cramping
■ Abdominal distention	■ Abdominal distention
■ Nausea and early, profuse vomiting	■ Minimal or no vomiting (vomiting may contain fecal material)
■ Obstipation	■ Obstipation
■ Severe fluid and electrolyte imbalances	■ No major fluid and electrolyte imbalances
■ Metabolic alkalosis	■ Metabolic acidosis

From *Medical-Surgical Nursing: A Nursing Process Approach* (p. 1613), by D. D. Ignatavicius, M. L. Workman, and M. A. Mishler, 1995, Philadelphia: W. B. Saunders. Reprinted with permission.

Manual disimpaction is usually required before an enema is administered; otherwise the solution will not be effective. An oil-retention enema followed by a sodium phosphate Fleets enema is often prescribed.

Diarrhea

Diarrhea is the opposite of constipation; it can be defined as frequent liquid or semisolid stools that are difficult to control. Chronic diarrhea may occur as part of a chronic bowel disease such as ulcerative colitis. Most commonly, though, nursing home residents tend to experience acute diarrhea.

FACTORS CONTRIBUTING TO DIARRHEA

Acute (noninfectious) diarrhea is usually a side effect of drug therapy, especially with antibiotics, or it may be the result of an enteric infection. Gastroenteritis associated with influenza or food is fairly common in nursing homes, where large numbers of residents are in close contact with each other or eat food prepared in a common kitchen.

Another type of infection is an indirect result of antibiotic therapy. When elderly or otherwise immunocompromised residents receive antibiotics, the normal flora of the bowel diminishes, giving rise to infectious pathogens, such as *Clostridium difficile (C. difficile).*

Regardless of the cause, diarrhea, especially in elderly residents, can be life-threatening. Residents can become rapidly dehydrated and develop severe electrolyte imbalances.

ASSESSMENT OF RESIDENTS WITH DIARRHEA

The daily record of stools alerts the nurse that the resident has diarrhea. As mentioned previously in this chapter under "Constipation," diarrheal stools may be caused by impaction. If the impaction is low, a digital examination can confirm the impaction.

In addition to the daily record of stools, the nurse notes whether the resident has begun a new drug, especially antibiotic therapy. If the stools have a very foul odor, *C. difficile* may be present. A stool culture may detect any pathogenic etiology for the diarrhea.

The resident must also be observed for manifestations associated with dehydration and electrolyte imbalances (e.g., sodium and potassium), particularly fever, weakness, and decreased mental status. Chapter 6 describes specific fluid and electrolyte imbalances in detail.

INTERVENTIONS FOR RESIDENTS WITH DIARRHEA

The most important intervention for residents with diarrhea is fluid administration to prevent dehydration. For severe diarrhea, oral rehydration therapy (ORT) is the most cost-effective method for fluid replacement. Commercial solutions that are specifically formulated to replace electrolytes as well as fluids should be used to replace losses from diarrhea liter for liter, especially for elderly residents. Resol, Ricelyte, and Rehydralyte are examples of solutions that can be used. Residents experiencing severe dehydration may require intravenous rehydration.

To minimize the number of stools, antidiarrheal agents, such as Kaopectate or Loperamide (Imodium), can be administered. However, these drugs should only be used in residents with noninfectious diarrhea. For infectious diarrhea, the preferred treatment is a course of an appropriate anti-infective drug to combat the causative agent. Metronidazole (Flagyl) and vancomycin (Vancocin) are commonly used drugs for *C. difficile*. Most residents require intravenous drug therapy followed by oral medication.

Residents with infectious diarrhea need to be removed from other residents to prevent the spread of the organism. Meticulous handwashing and infection control techniques are vital. Some states require that admissions, visitors, and daily recreational activities be suspended until the residents recover.

One of the biggest issues surrounding *C. difficile* infections is determining when the resident can be readmitted to the nursing home if she or he has been hospitalized for the infection. Some nursing homes have a policy that the resident must have a negative stool culture before readmission. This policy is unrealistic because some residents will continue to colonize the pathogen. If the resident no longer has diarrhea, he or she can safely return to the facility after treatment. If symptoms recur, the resident has a repeat infection and must be treated.

Any resident with diarrhea is at high risk for skin breakdown. Most residents with diarrhea are incontinent because the diarrhea makes elimination difficult to control. Keeping the skin dry and clean is essential. Protective, moisture-proof cremes applied after every cleansing can be especially helpful.

CHAPTER HIGHLIGHTS

Multiple physiologic and environmental factors place the elderly resident at high risk for falls.

If a resident falls, the nurse assesses level of conciousness to determine the presence of a head injury; hip fracture is also a common result of a fall.

The Braden and Norton scales are excellent assessment tools for determining a resident's risk of developing pressure ulcers.

Pressure ulcers are staged as I (reddened skin that does not blanch) through IV (skin broken and ulcer extending into muscle or possibly bone).

The five types of chronic urinary incontinence are stress, overflow, urge, functional, and mixed incontinence.

The three common mental health problems among the elderly are depression, delirium, and dementia; depression is the most common.

Alzheimer's disease is the most common dementia occurring in the elderly.

Environmental restructuring and managing difficult behaviors are important nursing interventions for the resident with dementia.

Undernutrition in the elderly can be assessed by weight and height, skin fold measurements, and laboratory tests, such as serum transferrin and albumin.

Enteral nutrition is preferred over parenteral nutrition because the resident's digestive tract is used.

The nurse must closely monitor the resident receiving either enteral or parenteral nutrition for complications associated with the solutions or administration systems.

Constipation is a very common problem among elderly; prevention focuses on high fiber in the diet, adequate fluids, and participation in exercise.

Diarrhea is also common in the elderly; *C. difficile* is an infectious diarrhea resulting from antibiotic administration.

Infectious diarrhea is treated with the appropriate antimicrobial drug; noninfectious diarrhea is treated with antidiarrheal medications to prevent dehydration.

REFERENCES AND READINGS

American Society of Parenteral and Enteral Nutrition (A.S.P.E.N.) (1993). Section II: Rationale for adult nutrition support guidelines. *Journal of Parenteral and Enteral Nutrition, 17*(4), 5SA–6SA.

Baker, S. P., & Harvey, A. H. (1985). Fall injuries in the elderly. *Clinical Geriatric Medicine, 1,* 501–525.

Beck, C. K., Heacock, P., Rapp, C. G., & Shue, V. (1993). Cognitive impairment in the elderly. *Nursing Clinics of North America, 28*(2), 335–348.

Beck, C. K., & Shue, V. M. (1994). Interventions for treating disruptive behavior in demented elderly people. *Nursing Clinics of North America, 29*(1), 143–156.

Bockus, S. (1993). When your patient needs tube feedings: Making the right decisions. *Nursing93, 23*(7), 34–43.

Booker, M. F., & Ignatavicius, D. D. (1996). *Infusion therapy: Techniques and medications.* Philadelphia: W. B. Saunders.

Bosek, M. S. D. & Savage, T. A. (1995). Ethics. In D. D. Ignatavicius, M. L. Workman, & M. A. Mishler (Eds.), *Medical-surgical nursing: A nursing process approach* (pp. 81–100). Philadelphia: W. B. Saunders.

Braun, J. V., & Lipson, S. (1993). *Toward a restraint free environment.* Baltimore: Health Professions Press.

Brown, M. K., & Everett, I. (1990). Gentler bowel fitness with fiber. *Geriatric Nursing, 11*(1), 26–27.

Buckwalter, K. C., & Babich, K. S. (1990). Psychologic and physiologic aspects of depression. *Nursing Clinics of North America, 25*(4), 945–954.

Cella, M. (1988). The nursing costs of urinary incontinence in a nursing home population. *Nursing Clinics of North America, 23*(1), 159–168.

Colburn, L. (1990). Preventing pressure ulcers: How to recognize and care for patients at risk. *Nursing90, 20*(2), 60–63.

Cuzzell, J. (1995). Interventions for clients with problems of the skin and nails. In D. D. Ignatavicius, M. L. Workman, & M. A. Mishler. *Medical-surgical nursing: A nursing process approach* (pp. 1929–1970). Philadelphia: W. B. Saunders.

De Keyser, G., Dejaeger, E., De Meyst, H., & Evers, G. C. M. (1994). Pressure-reducing effects of heel protectors. *Advances in Wound Care, 7*(4), 30–34.

Depression Guideline Panel. (1993). *Depression in primary care: Volume 2. Treatment of major depression. Clinical practice guideline, Number 5* (AHCPR Pub. No. 93-0551). Rockville, MD: U.S. Department of Health and Human Services, Public Health Service, Agency for Health Care Policy and Research.

Ebersole, P., & Hess, P. (1994). *Toward healthy aging: Human needs and nursing response.* St. Louis: Mosby.

Fater, K. H. (1995). Determining nasoenteral feeding tube placement. *MEDSURG Nursing, 4*(1), 27–32.

Feil, N. (1993). *Validation: The Feil method.* Cleveland, OH: Edward Feil Productions.

Fine, J. I., & Rouse-Bane, S. (1995). Using validation techniques to improve communication with cognitively impaired older adults. *Journal of Gerontological Nursing, 21*(6), 39–45.

Foreman, M. D. (1990). Complexities of acute confusion. *Geriatric Nursing, 11,* 136–139.

Frantz, R. A., & Ferrell-Torry, A. (1993). Physical impairments in the elderly population. *Nursing Clinics of North America, 28*(2), 363–372.

Funk, S. G., Tournquist, E. M., Champagne, M. T., & Wiese, R. A. (1992). *Key aspects of elder care: Managing falls, incontinence, and cognitive impairment.* New York: Springer.

Galindo-Ciocon, D. J., Ciocon, J. O., & Galindo, D. J. (1995). Gait training and falls in the elderly. *Journal of Gerontological Nursing, 21*(6), 10–18.

Haight, B. K. (1995). Suicide risk in frail elderly people relocated to nursing homes. *Geriatric Nursing, 16*(3), 104–107.

Hall, G. R. (1994). Caring for people with Alzheimer's disease using the conceptual model of progressively lowered stress threshold in the clinical setting. *Nursing Clinics of North America, 29*(1), 129–142.

Ignatavicius, D. D., Workman, M. L., & Mishler, M. A. (1995). *Medical-surgical nursing: A nursing process approach.* Philadelphia: W. B. Saunders.

Keane, S. M. & Sells, S. (1990). Recognizing depression in the elderly. *Journal of Gerontological Nursing, 16*(1), 21–25.

Kelly, L. S., & Mobily, P. (1991). Iatrogenesis in the elderly: Impaired skin integrity. *Journal of Gerontological Nursing, 17*(3), 24–29.

Knox, D. M., Anderson, T. M., & Anderson, P. S. (1994). Effects of different turn intervals on skin of healthy adults. *Advances in Wound Care, 7*(1), 48–56.

Krasner, D. (1995). Wound care: How to use the red-yellow-black system. *American Journal of Nursing, 95*(5), 44–47.

Kuehn, A. F., & Sendelweck, S. (1995). Acute health status and its relationship to falls in the nursing home. *Journal of Gerontological Nursing, 21*(7), 41–49.

Lee, C. A., Barrett, A., & Ignatavicius, D. D. (1996). *Stroot's fluids and electrolytes: A practical approach.* Philadelphia: F. A. Davis.

Lord L. M., Lipp, J., & Stull, S. (1996). Adult tube feeding formulas. *MEDSURG Nursing: The Journal of Adult Health, 5*, 407–421.

Mahan, L. K., & Arlin, M. (1992). *Krause's food, nutrition, and diet therapy.* Philadelphia: W. B. Saunders.

Manion, P. S., & Rantz, M. J. (1995). Relocation stress syndrome: A comprehensive plan for long-term care admissions. *Geriatric Nursing, 16*(3), 108–112.

Mentes, J. C. (1995). A nursing protocol to assess causes of delirium. *Journal of Gerontological Nursing, 21*(2), 26–30.

Miller, C. A. (1995). Decisions about behavior-modifying medications for people with dementia. *Geriatric Nursing, 16*(3), 143–144.

Miller, D., & Miller, H. W. (1995). Giving meds through the tube. *RN, 58*(1), 44–47.

National Institute on Aging. (1990). *Special report on aging.* Rockville, MD: U.S. Department of Health and Human Services. Public Health Service.

National Institutes of Health. (1990). Urinary incontinence in adults; Consensus conference. *Journal of the American Medical Association, 261*, 2685.

Panel for the Prediction and Prevention of Pressure Ulcers in Adults. (1992). *Pressure ulcers in adults: Prediction and prevention. Clinical practice guideline, Number 3* (AHCPR Pub. No. 92-0047). Rockville, MD: U.S. Department of Health and Human Services, Public Health Service, Agency for Health Care Policy and Research.

Powell, S. (1993). Restraint reduction: Customizing approaches to care. *Provider, 1*(2), 76–77.

Rader, J. (1993). Modifying the environment to decrease the use of restraints. *Journal of Gerontological Nursing, 17*(2), 9–13.

Ripich, D. N., Wykle, M., & Niles, S. (1995). Alzheimer's disease caregivers: The FOCUSED program. *Geriatric Nursing, 16*(1), 15–19.

Sambandham, M., & Schirm, V. (1995). Music as an intervention for residents with Alzheimer's disease in long-term care. *Geriatric Nursing, 16*(2), 84–88.

Shelton, S., & Ignatavicius, D. D. (1995). Interventions for clients with other nutritional problems. In D. D. Ignatavicius, M. L. Workman, & M. A. Mishler (Eds.). *Medical-surgical nursing: A nursing process approach* (pp. 1761–1782). Philadelphia: W. B. Saunders.

Snyder, M., Egan, E. C., & Burns, K. R. (1995). Interventions for decreasing agitation in persons with dementia. *Journal of Gerontogical Nursing, 21*(7), 34–40.

Stanley, M., & Beare, P. G. (1995). *Gerontological nursing.* Philadelphia: F. A. Davis.

Steiner, D., & Marcopulos, B. (1991). Depression in the elderly: Characteristics and clinical management. *Nursing Clinics of North America, 26*(3), 585–600.

Sturm, R., & Wells, K. B. (1995). How can care for depression become more cost-effective? *Journal of the American Medical Association, 273*, 51–58.

Tideiksaar, R. (1993). *Falls in older persons: Prevention and management in hospitals and nursing homes.* Denver, Colorado: Tactilitics.

Tinetti, M. E., & Speechley, M. (1990). Prevention of falls among the elderly. *New England Journal of Medicine, 320*, 1055–1059.

Urinary Incontinence Guideline Panel. (1992). *Urinary incontinence in adults. Clinical practice guideline* (AHCPR Pub. No. 92-0038). Rockville, MD: U.S. Department of Health and Human Services, Public Health Service, Agency for Health Care Policy and Research.

Viall, C. (1995). Taking the mystery out of TPN. *Nursing95, 25*(4), 34–43.

Webber-Jones, J., et al. (1992). How to declog a feeding tube. *Nursing92, 22*(4), 62–64.

Weick, M. D. (1992). Physical restraints? An FDA update. *American Journal of Nursing, 92*(8), 102–103.

Weinstein, S. M. (1993). *Plumer's principles and practice of intravenous therapy.* Philadelphia: W. B. Saunders.

Woods, P., & Ashley, J. (1995). Simulated presence therapy: Using selected memories to manage problem behaviors in Alzheimer's disease patients. *Geriatric Nursing, 16*(1), 9–14.

Yakabowich, M. (1990). Prescribe with care: The role of laxatives in the treatment of constipation. *Journal of Gerontological Nursing, 16*(7), 4–11.

Yazdanfar, D. J. (1990). Assessing the mental status of the cognitively impaired elderly. *Journal of Gerontological Nursing, 16*(9), 32–36.

Yen, P. K. (1995). Digestive dilemmas. *Geriatric nursing, 16*(3), 141–142.

Young, E. M. (1989). *Geriatric dermatology: Clinical diagnosis and practical therapy.* New York: Igaku-Shoin.

DISCUSSION QUESTIONS TO PROMOTE CRITICAL THINKING

1. A resident has two blackened, discolored heels. How should this skin change be staged?

2. What type of activities would be appropriate for the client with middle stage Alzheimer's disease?

3. A resident diagnosed with depression has been on antidepressant medication for 5 days. The family wants to know why the resident has not improved. What is the probable explanation for this observation?

4. One of your geriatric nursing assistants places a brief on an incontinent resident while in bed. You asked the assitant to use underpads instead of the brief while the resident is in bed, but she doesn't understand the rationale for your request. How would you explain it to her?

5 Medication Use in the Elderly

OUTLINE

Factors Contributing to Multiple Drug Use Among the Elderly

Pharmacokinetics and the Elderly

Common Complications of Drug Therapy in the Elderly

Pain Management in the Elderly

Infusion Therapy in Nursing Homes

Unnecessary Drugs

Self-Administration of Drugs

Administering Tips for Medication

OBJECTIVES

- Identify factors contributing to multiple drug use among the elderly
- Identify common physiologic changes and diseases that can affect drug use in the elderly
- Describe nursing considerations for pain management in the elderly
- Discuss nursing interventions for elderly residents receiving intravenous therapy

Although the elderly represent only about 13 percent of the United States population, they use more than one-third of all prescription medications. They also consume more than one-third of all over-the-counter (OTC) drugs, especially acetaminophen (Tylenol), aspirin, laxatives, antacids, and vitamins. This multiple drug use among the elderly population is often referred to as "polypharmacy."

Factors Contributing to Multiple Drug Use Among the Elderly

A number of factors contribute to multiple drug use among the elderly:

1. A high incidence of chronic illness
2. Self-medication
3. The use of drugs to treat side effects of other drugs
4. The lack of education among health care providers (physicians, physician assistants, and nurse practitioners) about the use of drugs for people older than 65 years.

First, as one ages, the incidence of chronic illness increases. Most people over 65 years of age take at least one prescribed medication for chronic illness, such as diabetes, heart disease, or arthritis. Medication is often the most cost-effective way to treat age-related health problems.

In addition to prescribed drugs, many elders self-medicate with OTC drugs when they have a health problem rather than consult a physician. The cost or fear of health care may keep them from seeking professional health services. Aches and pains associated with arthritis may be self-treated with acetaminophen or aspirin. Indigestion and constipation, two common gastrointestinal problems associated with aging, may be treated with OTC antacids and laxatives. Vitamins may be consumed to help meet basic nutritional needs in older adults who have a poor appetite.

A common practice that compounds the polypharmacy problem is the tendency of many elderly to consult a variety of sources for health care and medications. These sources include friends, family, and numerous pharmacies and physicians. This practice can result in duplication of medications. For instance, an individual may be taking prescribed ibuprofen (Motrin) for arthritis but taking OTC ibuprofen, such as Advil, on the advice of a friend. The result can be an ibuprofen overdose with serious adverse effects.

Because drug side effects are most common in the over-65 age group, additional drugs may be prescribed to combat these undesired effects. For example, it is very common for an elder to be receiving furosemide (Lasix) for congestive heart failure and potassium supplements to prevent or treat hypokalemia (decreased serum potassium) associated with furosemide therapy. An oral hypoglycemic may be needed to control blood glucose in an individual who is on prednisone (Deltasone) for chronic airflow limitation (CAL) (also called chronic obstructive pulmonary disease, or COPD).

Probably the most important factor that contributes to multiple drug use is the lack of education among health care providers about elder care and medication use in the elderly. As discussed in the next section of this chapter, the physiologic changes associated with aging markedly affect the way that drugs are used in the body. Drug manufacturers do not routinely recommend dosing schedules for individuals older than 65 years or specify over what period of time each drug should be administered.

Physicians tend to keep their elderly clients on the same medications for a long period of time, then add other medications to the regimen as new health problems arise. In hospitals and nursing homes, clinical pharmacists often review the drug regimen and assist the physician in identifying potential problems with drug therapy. As the number of board-certified geriatricians and geriatric nurse practitioners increases, drugs for the elderly will be more carefully prescribed and monitored.

The results of multiple drug use among the elderly are serious adverse effects or death. One in five elder admissions to a hospital is caused by adverse drug reactions, especially related to the use of aspirin, diuretics, analgesics, digoxin, prednisone, and warfarin (Coumadin). When five drugs are used, the risk of adverse effects is 50 percent; when eight or more drugs are used, the risk is 100 percent. The average number of prescribed medications for nursing home residents is seven to eight.

Nurses caring for older adults in any setting need to educate them about the need to seek professional medical advice before taking any prescribed or OTC drug. Elders who attend senior citizens' centers or live in retirement communities are often exposed to educational programs about drug therapy in the elderly. Some centers routinely assess each participant's current drug regimen by asking elders to bring all of their medications to the nurse or pharmacist for evaluation. Some large pharmacies in the community also offer this service. Most community pharmacies are also able to track medication profiles for their customers and provide consumer education to help prevent negative outcomes.

Nurses who work in nursing homes and other health care agencies should also take a drug history to determine what medications the resident has been taking. If the resident is unable to provide the information, the nurse can ask the family or significant other to recall or bring in the medications that the resident was taking, both prescribed and over-the-counter drugs.

Pharmacokinetics and the Elderly

As discussed in Chapter 3, numerous physiologic changes occur during the aging process. Many of these changes negatively affect the pharmacokinetics of medication, that is, the way that a drug is absorbed, distributed and used, metabolized, and excreted by the body. In addition to normal physiologic changes experienced by many elders, chronic diseases and illnesses can interfere with pharmacokinetics as well. Table 5–1 summarizes some of the most common physiologic changes and diseases that can affect drug use in the elderly.

DRUG ABSORPTION

As one ages, the motility of the digestive tract slows, a change whose result is a delayed emptying by the stomach. Therefore, oral drugs take longer to move into the small intestine and be absorbed through the intestinal mucosa then in a younger person.

Absorption of injectables may also be affected, because blood flow to subcutaneous and muscle tissue decreases with aging. In a thin elderly person, inadequate subcutaneous tissue may prevent proper administration of insulin or heparin.

In addition to the typical physiologic changes of the gastrointestinal tract, many elders experience diseases of the "gut," such as malabsorption syndrome, inflammatory bowel disease (colitis), or diverticulosis. These disorders decrease the ability of drugs to be absorbed into the bloodstream for use by the body.

DRUG DISTRIBUTION

Once a drug is absorbed, it must be carried by the bloodstream for use throughout the body. As one ages, blood circulation diminishes and the amount of body water decreases, resulting in lower blood volume for transporting medication. In older adults who become undernourished,

Table 5–1. **Common Physiologic Changes and Diseases That Can Affect Drug Use in the Elderly**

	Physiologic Changes	**Diseases**
Drug Absorption	Decreased gastrointestinal motility Delayed stomach emptying Decreased stomach acids Decreased subcutaneous tissue Diminished blood flow to skin and gut	Malabsorption syndrome Inflammatory bowel disease Malnutrition
Drug Distribution	Decreased body water Decreased circulation	Malnutrition (low albumin)
Drug Metabolism	Decreased blood flow to liver Diminished liver function	Cirrhosis Chronic hepatitis
Drug Excretion	Diminished renal function Decreased creatinine clearance	Chronic renal failure

serum albumin (protein) levels fall. Many drugs are highly protein-bound and can only be distributed and used by the body if they are bound to albumin. Table 5–2 lists some of the most common protein-binding drugs. Serum albumin levels must be carefully monitored in elders, especially those receiving any protein-binding drug. If the albumin falls below 3.2 g/L, protein intake through the diet or supplements should be increased.

DRUG METABOLISM

Most drugs are metabolized by the liver. Put simply, in this process the liver breaks down drugs so that they can be safely used by the body. As one ages, decreased blood flow to the liver slows the ability of the liver to metabolize drugs. The result is that the half-life of the drug (the time for the drug plasma level to be reduced by half) increases. In other words, drugs in an elderly person tend to "hang around" longer in their toxic, nonmetabolized form. The problem is worsened in an individual who has liver disease, such as cirrhosis or chronic hepatitis.

DRUG EXCRETION

Probably the most important cause of adverse and toxic effects associated with drug therapy in the elderly is diminished kidney function. Almost all drugs and their metabolites are excreted by the kidneys. But, as described in Chapter 3, kidney function markedly declines as one ages, by as much as 50 percent or more. The result is a buildup of drugs in the body that can lead to serious toxicities, even death. If the older adult has renal disease, the problem is compounded.

Common Complications of Drug Therapy in the Elderly

As a result of multiple drug use in the elderly and the physiologic changes associated with the aging process, the older adult is predisposed to many

Table 5–2. **Common Protein-Binding Drugs**

Aspirin	Warfarin (Coumadin)
Ibuprofen (Motrin)	Phenytoin (Dilantin)
Sulindac (Clinoril)	Furosemide (Lasix)
Indomethacin (Indocin)	Haloperidol (Haldol)
Naproxen (Naprosyn)	Chlorothiazide (Diuril)
Tolbutamide (Orinase)	Verapamil (Calan)
Chlorpropamide (Diabenese)	Nifedipine (Procardia)

complications of drug therapy, especially adverse effects, including toxicities and death.

To help minimize drug complications, dosing must be carefully considered. Although no specific guidelines for dosing have been established, the "rule of thumb" for prescribing medications for the elderly is "start low, go slow." This guideline means that the lowest possible dose of the medication should be tried. If the drug is effective, the dose does not need to be increased. If it is not effective, the dose should be increased *gradually* in small increments.

While physicians, physician assistants, and nurse practitioners are responsible for *prescribing* medications in the nursing home setting, nurses have responsibilities regarding drug therapy as well. Of primary importance is the need for nurses to have a broad knowledge base about the polypharmacy problem in the elderly and specific nursing interventions to prevent, minimize, and monitor drug use in the elderly.

Nurses should also be aware of both the desired therapeutic effects and the unwanted adverse effects of the medications they administer. In some cases, adverse effects can be avoided or detected early through careful assessment. For example, diminished renal function as a consequence of antibiotic therapy may be detected by assessing urinary output and by monitoring serum creatinine and blood urea nitrogen (BUN) levels. When adverse effects are suspected, the nurse should discontinue the offending medication and notify the health care provider. Table 5–3 lists some drugs typically used for the elderly, together with common adverse effects. The nurse should monitor for and report these problems.

Table 5–3. Common Adverse Effects of Major Drugs Used for the Elderly

Drug Classification	Adverse Effects
Diuretics	Dehydration, hypokalemia, hyponatremia
Corticosteroids	Fluid overload, hypernatremia, hypokalemia, hyperglycemia, osteoporosis, GI ulcers
Antibiotics (especially aminoglycosides)	Renal failure
Digitalis preparations	Dysrhythmias, depression
Antipsychotics	Anticholinergic effects, such as dry mouth, constipation, urinary retention, blurred vision; confusion; sedation; tardive dyskinesia (irreversible)
Antidepressants	Anorexia, anticholinergic effects; weight loss, sedation
Nonsteroidal anti-inflammatory agents	Bleeding, GI ulcers, tinnitus
Oral hypoglycemic agents	Liver dysfunction
Opioid analgesics	Sedation, respiratory depression, constipation, psychoses (meperidine [Demerol])
Antihypertensive agents	Depression, orthostatic hypotension

Pain Management in the Elderly

One of the most important aspects of elder care related to medication administration is the management of acute and chronic pain. Despite numerous alternatives to drug therapy for pain management, such as massage, imagery, positioning, ice, and heat, medications are frequently required to help relieve pain. A combination of pharamcologic and non-pharmacologic measures can help reduce the amount of pain medication needed, depending on the individual.

For years, nurses and physicians have been taught to be extremely cautious about opioid (narcotic) administration for people over 65 because opioids can cause respiratory depression and sedation in this group. The result of this message is that health professionals actually *undermedicate* the elderly who are experiencing pain, causing them needless suffering and a poor quality of life (Behrens, 1996; Hill, 1990; Haviley et al., 1992). In addition, most health care professionals have not been taught how to accurately assess a person's pain level and how to distinguish types of pain.

DEFINITIONS AND PERCEPTIONS OF PAIN

A number of definitions of pain are found in the literature, but no one definition is more accepted than another. The International Association on Pain (1979) defined pain as an unpleasant sensory and emotional experience associated with tissue damage. This definition includes both the physiologic and psychologic (emotional) aspects of pain.

Margo McCaffery (1979), a nurse who specializes in pain assessment and management, provides a more personal explanation of pain: "Pain is whatever the experiencing person says it is and exists whenever he says it does" (p. 11). This definition indicates that pain is very subjective. This subjectivity limits the health professional's understanding of the person's perception (feelings) of and response to pain. Several factors seem to influence pain perception, including age, gender, and culture.

Experts agree that pain perception in the older adult differs from that of younger adults. However, the exact nature of the difference is not clear. The perception of cutaneous (skin) pain may decrease due to physiologic changes in the skin associated with aging, such as a diminished blood supply. The perception of visceral (organ) pain may actually increase in older adults (Egbert, 1991; Neeley, 1993).

Older adults tend to report complaints of pain less often than their younger counterparts, which may explain why they receive less analgesics (pain medications) or are thought to experience less pain as they age. Neeley (1993) describes the following beliefs and concerns that most elderly individuals have about pain:

- Moderate or severe pain indicates a serious illness or impending death.

- Mild pain is something that they must learn to live with as a part of the aging process.

- Expressing pain is not acceptable and is a sign of weakness.

- Nurses are too busy to listen to complaints of pain.

- Complaining of pain will cause the staff to label the elder as a "bad" or "difficult" person.

- Opioid analgesics (narcotics) should be avoided because they are addictive.

By keeping these beliefs in mind, the nurse can educate the elderly individual about the need to report pain and receive mesaures that relieve the pain, including medication. The nurse needs to reassure elders that they will not be labeled in any negative way and that opioids are rarely addictive.

Gender may also influence one's interpretation and feelings about pain. Research has shown that nurses expect men to be more tolerant of pain than women. Women are expected to react more emotionally than men to pain (Walding, 1991). Research is also underway to establish how women and men differ in their response to all types of medication, including analgesics.

Transcultural Considerations in Assessing Pain

Only recently has these been consideration or study of transcultural variables as they affect pain perception or management. Some studies have found that there are no differences among cultures regarding pain perception (Gaston-Johansson et al., 1990; Zatzick & Dimsdale, 1990). However, people may express their pain in various ways. For example, Mexican-American women typically moan or cry when they are uncomfortable. Nurses who believe that these behaviors are not necessary may view these individuals negatively. These behaviors, though, may actually serve to help relieve pain rather than serve as an expression of pain (Calvillo & Flaskerud, 1991).

TYPES OF PAIN

To determine what interventions are needed to relieve pain, the type of pain that a person is experiencing must be assessed. Pain is usually categorized into two basic types—acute pain and chronic pain.

Acute Pain

Acute pain is typically temporary and occurs suddenly, such as the chest pain experienced during an angina attack. The individual having the pain can usually describe the nature of the pain, such as stabbing, crushing, throbbing, and so forth. The pain can also be localized such that the person can point to an area of the body where the pain occurs. As the affected tissues heal, the pain usually subsides.

Acute pain serves a biologic purpose because it acts as a warning signal to the body that a problem exists. Acute pain alerts the sympathetic nervous system ("fight-or-flight"), which increases the level of serum epinephrine (adrenaline) and norepinephrine. These hormones cause rapid responses in the body, including an increased heart rate, blood pressure, and respiratory rate; sweating; and dilated pupils. Restlessness, anxiety, and apprehension are also common.

Postoperative pain is one of the most common types of acute pain. According to the Acute Pain Management Guideline Panel (1992), many postoperative clients do not receive adequate analgesia to relieve their pain. Pain does not subside until the affected body tissues have healed, often 6 weeks or longer after surgery.

Chronic Pain

Chronic pain is not well understood. Over 25 percent of people in the United States, most over 65 years old, have chronic pain (Polomano & Ignatavicius, 1995). Chronic pain typically lasts for more than 6 months, has a gradual onset, and is difficult to localize. The sympathetic responses associated with acute pain are not present in individuals with chronic pain.

Chronic pain can be the result of a number of illnesses or trauma. In general, it is divided into chronic malignant (cancer-related) pain and chronic nonmalignant pain, pain resulting from causes other than cancer, such as arthritis. Because chronic pain lasts for an extended period of time, it tends to interfere with the ability of an individual to function and maintain a high quality of life. Table 5–4 compares and contrasts the physiologic and behavioral responses to acute and chronic pain.

ASSESSMENT OF PAIN IN THE ELDERLY

A variety of pain assessment tools are cited in the literature, some very simple and some more complex. In a nursing home setting, the nurse needs to make an accurate but time-efficient assessment of the resident's pain. Noting the resident's response, both physiologic and behavioral, can help the nurse determine the type of pain—acute or chronic—that is present.

The P-Q-R-S-T model can be very useful in obtaining a comprehensive assessment of the resident's pain:

P Provoking incident? (Was there a certain incident or event that caused the pain?)

Table 5–4. **Physiologic and Behavioral Responses to Acute and Chronic Pain**

Pain Type	Physiologic Response	Behavioral Response
Acute	▪ Increased blood pressure initially ▪ Increased pulse rate ▪ Increased respiratory rate ▪ Dilated pupils ▪ Perspiration	▪ Restlessness ▪ Inability to concentrate ▪ Apprehension ▪ Distress
Chronic	▪ Normal blood pressure ▪ Normal pulse rate ▪ Normal respiratory rate ▪ Normal pupils ▪ Dry skin	▪ Immobility or physical inactivity ▪ Withdrawal ▪ Despair

From *Medical-Surgical Nursing: A Nursing Process Approach* (p. 127), by D. D. Ignatavicius, M. L. Workman, and M. A. Mishler, 1995, Philadelphia: W. B. Saunders. Reprinted with permission.

Q Quality of pain? (What does the pain feel like to the resident? Is it burning, stabbing, crushing, throbbing, etc.?)

R Region, radiation, and relief? (Where is the pain located and does it radiate, or travel? Does anything help the pain?)

S Severity of pain? (How severe is the pain? On a scale of 1 to 5 with 5 being the worst, describe the pain.)

T Time? (How long does the pain last and when does it occur?)

If the resident is not able to communicate or is confused, this assessment model is not appropriate. The nurse then needs to rely on other indicators of pain such as nonverbal cues. Is the resident grimacing or guarding an area of the body? Is the resident restless or exhibiting emotional behaviors, such as severe agitation or screaming? When residents in nursing homes manifest emotional behaviors, they may be diagnosed as demented and then given psychotropic medications to sedate them rather than pain medication to relieve their pain.

INTERVENTIONS FOR PAIN MANAGEMENT IN THE ELDERLY

Drug Therapy

Pain management requires an interdisciplinary approach. Each member of the health team must advocate for residents when they are not able to make their needs known. If the resident cannot communicate, the staff must anticipate the resident's need for pain relief. For example, residents with fractured hip repair are typically admitted to a nursing home or transitional care unit for rehabilitation between the 4th and 6th postoperative day (or earlier). In the hospital, the resident received oral opioid analgesics for pain relief. In the nursing home, the physician's orders may include only acetaminophen (Tylenol) as needed for pain. The resident becomes restless and agitated because bone pain is very uncomfortable and the tissues affected by surgery have not had time to heal. The nurse must advocate for the resident and obtain an order for a stronger analgesic for unrelieved pain.

In general, oral pain medications are preferred over parenterals because they are less invasive and tend to be better absorbed by older adults. Many people underestimate the effectiveness of nonopioid analgesics for chronic pain or mild acute pain. Nonsteroidal anti-inflammatory drugs, such as ibuprofen (Motrin), may be very effective in treating arthritis pain. Ketorolac (Toradol) may be very effective for short-term use in treating residents with acute pain.

Meperidine (Demerol), commonly used for acute postoperative pain, should not be used for elderly residents because it can cause severe adverse effects, such as seizures, hallucinations, and memory loss (Acute Pain Management Guideline Panel, 1992). Morphine and hydromorphone (Dilaudid) are the preferred drugs for acute postoperative pain when the parenteral route must be used.

Potent opioid analgesia is currently available in oral form for cancer pain, such as MS Contin. Transdermal (topical patch) fentanyl (Duragesic) is available in assorted strengths and can be easily administered in the nursing home setting for cancer pain. Adjuvant drugs, such as antidepressants, are also fairly commonly given for chronic pain.

In traditional nursing homes where intravenous therapy is used, or in subacute units, additional options for pain management may be available. These options include the patient-controlled analgesia (PCA) pump, continuous subcutaneous opioid analgesia, continuous intravenous opioid analgesia, and long-term intraspinal analgesia. It is not within the scope of this chapter to describe these systems in detail. Most are used for residents who have cancer pain that cannot be controlled by either the oral or topical routes (Booker & Ignatavicius, 1996).

Nonpharmacologic Interventions

Many nonpharmacologic interventions for pain management are described in the literature, such as biofeedback, imagery, hypnosis, and transelectric nerve stimulation (TENS). While these methods are often effective in managing pain in people who are cognitively intact, many elderly residents in nursing homes are not able to actively participate in their care and therefore cannot benefit from these measures.

Basic comfort measures can be helpful in reducing most types of pain. The severely arthritic resident usually benefits from the heat of a warm bath or shower early in the day. The resident whose painful knee has swollen from physical therapy after a total knee replacement may find relief with an ice pack.

Repositioning a painful part of the body may also be beneficial. Residents who have amputatations typically find that frequent repositioning can help with incisional pain and phantom limb pain, although drug therapy may also be needed. Many residents have increased pain at night because they no longer have the distractions of the daytime to keep their minds off their pain.

At bedtime, a backrub and warm beverage can assist in relaxing the resident. If not contraindicated, a small amount of an alcoholic liquer or glass of wine may relax the resident and promote rest.

Infusion Therapy in Nursing Homes

While many nursing homes do not provide infusion therapy, this trend is changing, especially with the growth of subacute care (see Chapter 9). Intravenous therapy is the most commonly administered type of infusion therapy in long term care facilities. While it is not within the scope of this chapter to discuss every aspect of infusion therapy, special considerations related to care of residents in the nursing home setting are described.

PURPOSES OF INFUSION THERAPY

The two most common purposes of infusion therapy in a nursing home are hydration and antibiotic therapy. Historically, when a nursing home resident became dehydrated or needed intravenous antibiotics for pneumonia or other acute infection, the resident was sent to a hospital. As discussed earlier in this book, relocating an elderly person who is ill can be very upsetting and result in acute confusion. By providing intravenous therapy in the facility, the resident can remain in the nursing home for treatment.

Hydration Therapy

Intravenous hydration usually requires several liters of isotonic or hypertonic fluid to replace body water and, in some cases, electrolytes. Isotonic solutions, such as 0.9 percent (normal) saline or 5 percent dextrose in water, provide the same osmolarity (concentration, or "pulling force") as the blood. Hypertonic solutions, such as 5 percent dextrose in 0.45 percent (½N) saline, have a higher osmolarity than blood and tend to pull water from the interstitial tissues of the body into the bloodstream (Table 5–5). The nurse's primary responsibility when caring for a resident receiving

Table 5–5. **Tonicity of Commonly Used Intravenous Solutions**

Solution	Tonicity
0.45% saline (½NS)	Hypotonic
0.9% saline (NS)	Isotonic
5% dextrose in water (5%D/W)	Isotonic
10% dextrose in water (10%D/W)	Hypertonic
5% dextrose in 0.9% saline (5%D/NS)	Hypertonic
5% dextrose in 0.45% saline (5%D/½NS)	Hypertonic
5% dextrose in 0.225% saline (5%D/¼NS)	Isotonic
Lactated Ringer's solution (RL)	Isotonic
5% dextrose in lactated Ringer's solution	Hypertonic

From *Stroot's Fluids and Electrolytes: A Practical Approach* (p. 207), by C. A. Lee, A. Barrett, and D. D. Ignatavicius, 1996, Philadelphia: F. A. Davis. Reprinted with permission.

intravenous therapy is to monitor for fluid and electrolyte imbalances, as discussed in Chapter 6.

Antibiotic Therapy

The development of increasingly potent oral antibiotics has reduced the need for intravenous antibiotic therapy. Antibiotics in any form should be administered with extreme caution in the elderly because they cause severe adverse effects, including kidney failure and death.

The long term care facility should have clear, updated policies regarding the definition of an infection and how it should be treated. For example, many nursing home residents colonize bacteria in their urine and have over 100,000 colonies present. In the past, the nurse reported this culture and sensitivity (C&S) finding to the physician, who would then place the resident on an antibiotic for a certain number of days. Current practice recognizes that unless the resident becomes symptomatic, he or she does not have a urinary tract infection and should therefore not be treated.

Keeping these newer practices in mind, it is not surprising that intravenous antibiotic therapy is not very common in the nursing home setting. Certain pneumonias and other acute infections, however, may require intravenous antibiotics via an intermittent infusion device (saline lock) or "piggybacked" into a continuous infusion providing hydration. As with any other medication, the nurse is responsible for correct drug administration and assessment for therapeutic and adverse effects. If the antibiotic is effective, the resident's temperature will return to baseline, and other signs and symptoms of infection will subside. In the event that the resident experiences an adverse effect, such as a rash or an elevated BUN and creatinine, the drug should be immediately discontinued and the health care provider should be notified.

Other Purposes

Pain Control

Occasionally the resident may need pain medication by an infusion route, as described earlier in this chapter. Continuous subcutaneous administration of opioid analgesics, usually morphine, via an electronic infusion device (pump) is the simplest and safest method for residents with terminal cancer. The nurse's primary responsibility when caring for a resident with either a patient-controlled device or a continuous infusion is to monitor for therapeutic and adverse effects of the medication. The resident may require other analgesics for "breakthrough" pain to supplement the infusion. Figure 5–1 shows an ambulatory pump that can be used for subcutaneous therapy.

Nutrition

Some residents, especially younger residents, may benefit from short-term parenteral nutrition rather than enteral nutrition. Partial parenteral nutrition (PPN) to supplement oral intake can be given through a peripheral (arm) intravenous access. However, total parenteral nutrition (TPN) can only be given through a central access device. Central access devices are long catheters that are generally placed into the superior vena cava or right atrium of the heart by a physician.

All parenteral nutrition solutions must be administered using an electronic infusion device due to the high amount of dextrose and other nutrients that are given. The nurse's primary responsibility when caring for a resident receiving either PPN or TPN is to monitor and report complications associated with therapy. The major complication is infection.

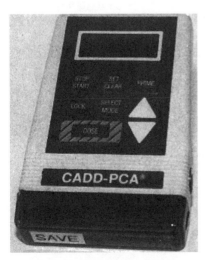

Figure 5–1. A continuous ambulatory drug delivery (CADD) pump used for infusion therapy. From *Infusion Therapy: Techniques and Medications* (p. 80), by M. Booker and D. D. Ignatavicius, 1996, Philadelphia: W. B. Saunders. Reprinted with permission.

Accurate vital sign assessment, especially temperature, is critical. Chapter 4 describes parenteral nutrition in detail.

INTERVENTIONS FOR THE ELDERLY RECEIVING INFUSION THERAPY

In facilities where infusion therapy is available, nurses need to be thoroughly educated in all aspects of care, including how to start the intravenous or subcutaneous therapy and how to manage the resident receiving the therapy. The elderly resident is at a special risk for complications associated with infusion therapy. The nurse needs to use adapted techniques when starting the intravenous "line" as well as minimize the risk of complications. For example, using a small gauge cannula and a blood pressure cuff as a tourniquet helps to minimize tissue trauma. Table 5–6 lists some of the most important nursing interventions for elderly residents receiving intravenous therapy.

Unnecessary Drugs

In October 1990, the federal Omnibus Budget Reconciliation Act (OBRA) was enacted to improve the quality of life of residents in nursing homes. One aspect of this landmark legislation addressed the polypharmacy problem in nursing homes. The law states that each resident's drug regimen must be "free of unnecessary drugs." An unnecessary drug is defined as any drug that is used:

Table 5–6. **Nursing Interventions for Elderly Residents Receiving Intravenous Therapy**

- Do not use regular tourniquets; use a blood pressure cuff instead.
- Use the shortest cannula or needle possible.
- Use the smallest gauge cannula or needle possible, unless blood is being administered.
- Do not tap the vein to "bring it up."
- Do not use the veins of the hand.
- Avoid large, tortuous superficial veins.
- Place the IV in the patient's lower forearm on the nondominant side unless the limb is weakened, traumatized, or paralyzed.
- Anchor the IV cannula with a transparent dressing unless the skin is exceptionally thin or the patient is taking corticosteroids.
- Use dry sterile gauze and wrap the arm loosely with gauze or flexible netting if the skin is thin and fragile; keep the puncture site exposed for assessment.
- Avoid restraints on the arm with the IV.
- Use electronic infusion devices or volume-controlled sets to prevent accidental fluid overload.
- Assess the IV site every 2–4 hours for complications.
- Maintain meticulous intake and output record.

From *Stroot's Fluids and Electrolytes: A Practical Approach* (p. 208), by C. A. Lee, A. Barrett, and D. D. Ignatavicius, 1996, Philadelphia: F. A. Davis. Reprinted with permission.

- In excessive doses
- For an excessively long time
- Without adequate monitoring for therapeutic and adverse effects
- Without adequate reason for the resident's being on the drug
- When adverse effects are present
- In any combination of the above reasons

This law has helped to decrease drug usage for nursing home residents by holding health care providers more accountable for their prescribing practices. The physician, physician assistant, or nurse practitioner must reevaluate each resident at least every 30 days for the need to continue with the drug regimen. The pharmacist must also periodically review each resident's drug profile and make recommendations to the health care provider for changes or monitoring strategies. For example, a resident receiving theophylline preparations must have frequent serum theophylline levels drawn to ensure that the resident is receiving the therapeutic amount.

Nurses also share the responsibility of carefully monitoring and documenting therapeutic and adverse effects. The OBRA legislation placed special emphasis on the use of antipsychotic drugs (see Table 4–8), often used to control behavioral manifestations associated with mental health or cognitive problems like dementia. The nurse uses a special medical record form to document these behaviors and any adverse effects of antipsychotic drugs. If no behaviors are present for several weeks or so, the drug dosage should be reduced. If the resident exhibits adverse effects, the drug dosage must be decreased or the drug must be discontinued, depending on the severity of the negative effect.

Self-Administration of Drugs

The OBRA legislation also allows the resident to self-administer medications *if* the interdisciplinary health team determines that this practice is safe. This issue is addressed as part of the interdisciplinary care plan. Very few elderly residents in nursing homes are able to give themselves their medication due to physical and/or cognitive problems. Younger residents are more likely able to self-medicate, but each resident must be evaluated for this ability.

Administering Tips for Medication

The majority of nursing homes residents are over 65 and experience both physiologic changes of aging and chronic illnesses that may compromise the ability of the nurse to administer medications. It takes time and patience to give medications to an elderly resident in a way that avoids choking and subsequent aspiration pneumonia.

Many residents have chewing or swallowing problems. For these individuals, crushing the medication and adding it to applesauce, pudding, or food of similar consistency can aid in the chewing and swallowing process. However, the nurse needs to make sure that the drug can be crushed. For example, slow-release drugs should *not* be crushed because the full dose will immediately be available for use by the body. Enteric-coated medications, such as Ecotrin, should not be crushed because they are designed to break down in the small intestine rather than in the stomach, where they can cause irritation.

Some residents do not need crushed medications, but they have difficulty swallowing large pills or capsules. Covering the medication with applesauce can facilitate the swallowing process. Liquid medications, unless they are thick, should be avoided when possible because they can cause aspiration.

Administration of medication through a feeding tube has already been disussed in Chapter 4.

When giving a subcutaneous injection, the nurse must find an area of the body with sufficient subcutaneous tissue to absorb the medication. Although the abdomen is the preferred site for heparin and insulin injections, it should not be used if the amount of subcutaneous tissue is not adequate. Other subcutaneous sites can be used for these medications if needed.

CHAPTER HIGHLIGHTS

Multiple drug use in the elderly is sometimes referred to as "polypharmacy."

Adverse effects of medication are much more common in older than in younger adults.

Physiologic changes associated with aging affect the way that drugs are absorbed, distributed, metabolized, and excreted by the body.

Health care providers and nurses typically undermedicate the elderly individual experiencing pain.

Pain management for the elderly requires an interdisciplinary team approach.

Elderly residents experience both acute and chronic pain. Acute pain stimulates the sympathetic nervous system, resulting in vital sign changes and sweating; chronic pain does not trigger this response, lasts more than 6 months, and causes a decline in quality of life.

The primary purposes of infusion therapy in nursing homes are hydration and antibiotic therapy.

The elderly resident receiving infusion therapy has special needs that must be considered.

The nurse is responsible for monitoring and documenting the therapeutic and adverse effects of medications.

The OBRA legislation mandated that residents of nursing homes must be free of unnecessary drugs and can self-administer their drugs if the practice is deemed safe by the interdisciplinary team.

REFERENCES AND READINGS

Acute Pain Management Guideline Panel. (1992). *Acute pain management: Operative or medical procedures and trauma. Clinical practice guideline.* AHCPR Pub. No. 92-0032. Rockville, MD: Agency for Health Care Policy and Research, Public Health Service, U.S. Department of Health and Human Services.

Alspach, G. (1994). Pain management: Dispelling some myths. *Critical Care Nurse, 5*, 13–15.

Behrens, E. (1996). An ethical approach to pain management. *MEDSURG Nursing: The Journal of Adult Health, 5*, 457–458.

Booker, M., & Ignatavicius, D. (1996). *Infusion therapy: Techniques and medications.* Philadelphia: W. B. Saunders.

Calvillo, E. R., & Flaskerud, J. H. (1991). Review of literature on culture and pain of adults with focus on Mexican-Americans. *Journal of Transcultural Nursing, 2*, 16–23.

Egbert, A. M. (1991). Help for the hurting elderly: Safe use of drugs to relieve pain. *Postgraduate Medicine, 89*(4), 217–228.

Gaston-Johansson, F., Albert, M., Fagan, E., & Zimmerman, L. (1990). Similarities in pain descriptions of four different ethnic-culture groups. *Journal of Pain and Symptom Management, 5*(2), 94–100.

Haviley, C., et al. (1992). Pharmacological management of cancer pain: A guide for the health professional. *Cancer Nursing, 15*, 331–346.

Hill, C. S., Jr. (1990). Relationship among cultural, educational, and regulatory agency influences on optimum cancer pain treatment. *Journal of Pain and Symptom Management, 5*(1) (Suppl.), S37–S45.

International Association on Pain, Mersky, H. (Chairman), Subcommittee on taxonomy. (1979). Pain terms: A list with definitions and notes on usage. *Pain, 6*, 249.

McCaffery, M. (1979). *Nursing management of the patient with pain.* Philadelphia: J. B. Lippincott.

Neeley, M. A. (1993). Pain management in elderly patients. *Med-Surg Nursing Quarterly, 1*(4), 32–51.

Polomano, R., & Ignatavicius, D. (1995). Pain. In D. D. Ignatavicius, M. L. Workman, & M. A. Mishler. *Medical-surgical nursing: A nursing process approach* (pp. 119–147). Philadelphia: W. B. Saunders.

Walding, M. F. (1991). Pain, anxiety, and powerlessness. *Journal of Advanced Nursing, 16*, 388–397.

Zalzick, D. F., & Dimsdale, J. E. (1990). Cultural variations in response to painful stimuli. *Psychosomatic Medicine, 52*, 544–557.

DISCUSSION QUESTIONS TO PROMOTE CRITICAL THINKING

1. Your nursing home unit admits a resident who has recently (5 days ago) undergone repair of a fractured hip. The physician ordered Tylenol tabs ii q4h PRN (every 4 hours, as needed) for incisional pain. The medication has not relieved the resident's pain. She is very restless and cries out when she is moved. What should your action be?

2. A resident was recently placed on a new antihypertensive medication. Since that time he has been more confused and at times combative. What adverse effect is he probably suffering from? What action should you take?

3. When helping a resident from the commode, you notice white powder in her stool. She has a history of malabsorption syndrome and colitis. What action should you take?

6

Acute Illnesses and Health Emergencies

OBJECTIVES

- Identify measures to prevent acute infections among nursing home residents
- Describe the physical assessment findings associated with fluid volume deficit and fluid overload
- Identify the common electrolyte imbalances seen in nursing home residents
- Differentiate diabetic ketoacidosis and hyperglycemia, hyperosmolar nonketotic syndrome
- State the atypical presentation of myocardial infarction in an elderly resident
- Compare and contrast the clinical manifestations of deep vein thrombosis and acute arterial occlusion

Nursing home residents of any age are at risk for acute illnesses and health emergencies. Some of the most common illnesses and emergencies are discussed in this chapter. The definition, prevention, assessment, and interventions for each problem are highlighted. The information in this chapter is not intended to be comprehensive. Additional information can be found in medical-surgical nursing textbooks. Chapter 4 describes emergencies, such as fractures and head injuries, that can result from falls.

Acute Infections

In the community, acute infections tend to occur most frequently in young and middle-aged adults, rather than in the elderly. However, acute infections are fairly common in nursing homes among all age groups due to the close proximity of residents and the number of visitors that come into these facilities.

The elderly in nursing homes tend to have multiple chronic illnesses that weaken and predispose them to acute infections. Another risk factor for infection in the elderly is the decline in the immune response associated with aging (see Chapter 3). The two most common infections seen among nursing home residents, especially the elderly, are respiratory infections and urinary tract infection.

RESPIRATORY INFECTIONS

The two major respiratory infections that affect nursing home residents are influenza and pneumonia.

Definitions

Influenza is a highly contagious, upper respiratory viral infection that occurs in people of all ages. The primary danger of influenza is that it can lead to complications, like pneumonia, which can be fatal.

In 1992, influenza and pneumonia were the sixth leading cause of death among all Americans, with a mortality rate of 31.8 per 100,000 people, and 89 percent of all deaths were in people over 65 years of age (Centers for Disease Control and Prevention, 1995).

Pneumonia is a lower respiratory tract infection that is often classified, on the basis of where the infection is acquired, as either community-acquired or nosocomial (hospital- or nursing home–acquired). Pneumonia is the second most common nosocomial infection seen among the hospitalized elderly.

Pneumonia may also be classified on the basis of its causative organism, most commonly bacteria or viruses. The elderly have a higher incidence of bacterial pneumonia than their younger counterparts. The most common pathogens causing pneumonia in nursing homes include *Streptococcus pneumoniae, Haemophilus influenzae, Klebsiella pneumoniae,* and influenza virus A or B (Cunha, Gingrich, & Rosebaum, 1990). If the nursing home resident acquires pneumonia during a hospital stay, *Klebsiella pneumoniae, Pseudomonas aeruginosa, Staphylococcus aureus,* and *Escherichia coli* are usually the causative pathogens (Fein, Feinsilver, & Niederman, 1991).

PREVENTION OF RESPIRATORY INFECTIONS

Prevention of pneumonia is a major goal for the health care team in the nursing home (Table 6–1). One of the most crucial measures for preventing pneumonia is identifying those residents who are most at risk. The elderly resident is typically more at risk than the younger resident. Other factors that increase the risk of acquiring pneumonia include tube feedings, poor nutritional state, intubation with a tracheostomy or endotracheal tube, smoking, prolonged immobility, tuberculosis, upper respiratory infection, and other chronic diseases.

Elderly residents who receive tube feedings, especially nasogastric (NG) feedings, are very predisposed to aspiration of the enteral formula. The NG tube diminishes the gag and cough reflexes, both of which usually serve as protection against aspiration. The formula can enter the lungs and provide a medium for bacterial growth, a condition referred to as *aspiration pneumonia.* This type of pneumonia can be deadly because it affects individuals who are already weak and possibly undernourished. Specific nursing interventions to prevent aspiration for residents who are tube-fed are discussed in Chapter 4 under the section on undernutrition.

Another vital measure in the prevention of pneumonia is the administration of influenza and pneumonia vaccines to residents 65 years of age and older and to residents who are immunocompromised, such as those with human immunodeficiency virus (HIV) infection. The influenza vaccine must be given annually because the causative viral strains vary from

Table 6–1. **Prevention of Pneumonia in the Nursing Home Resident**

- Identify high-risk residents, such as elderly, immobilized, and tube-fed residents.
- For tube-fed residents, take precautions to prevent aspiration, such as keeping the head of the resident's bed up at an angle of at least 30 degrees.
- Administer influenza and pneumonia vaccines.
- Teach residents to wash their hands frequently or assist the resident in washing hands.
- Keep healthy residents separated from those with infections.
- Remind residents to cover their mouths when coughing or sneezing, if possible.
- Keep residents adequately hydrated and in optimal nutritional health.

year to year. The pneumonia vaccine was intended as a once-in-a-lifetime vaccine. However, many physicians recommend revaccination every 5 to 7 years or depend upon serum titers to determine the need for another immunization.

All residents need adequate nutrition and hydration to help prevent respiratory infection. Healthy residents should be separated from those with highly contagious infections, many of which are spread through droplet or respiratory secretions.

Assessment

Diagnosis of respiratory infection in the elderly is often difficult because the classic signs and symptoms may be absent. The classic manifestations include fever, productive cough, chest discomfort, fatigue, dyspnea, and crackles. The white blood cell (WBC) count is typically elevated. Pneumonia is confirmed by the presence of infiltrates seen on x-ray. The causative organism is determined by sputum analysis.

Instead of the classic disease manifestations, the elderly usually display more vague signs and symptoms, which include confusion, fatigue, weakness, and decreased general functioning, all caused by decreased arterial oxygen. Fever and elevated WBCs are often absent or undetected because the elderly have a low oral temperature and a suppressed immune system (Matteson, McConnell, & Linton, 1997).

The nurse should carefully observe for changes in the resident's usual behavior and functioning and should suspect infection when significant behavioral changes occur.

Interventions

If respiratory infection is diagnosed early, the resident may be able to stay in the nursing home during treatment. Oral antimicrobial therapy may be sufficient for early or mild infection, but intravenous (IV) antibiotics are generally needed for residents with moderate to severe pneumonia. The type of drug prescribed depends on the type of pneumonia being treated.

All residents with respiratory infection need to rest and be adequately hydrated to reduce fever, if present, and to prevent dehydration. Continuous oxygen is typically used to improve ventilatory function and increase arterial oxygen levels. Breathing may also be facilitated by keeping the resident in a semi-Fowler position while in bed. For some residents, nebulizer treatments are used to administer medication directly into the lungs to open small airways and promote airflow.

The nurse monitors the resident's vital signs and WBC count and reports significant changes to the physician. Response to treatment is determined by periodic x-rays; the infiltrate should slowly resolve.

URINARY TRACT INFECTION

Urinary tract infections are very common among nursing home residents. The infection usually begins in the urethra and bladder and then may ascend into the kidneys if not treated.

Definition

One of the most important aspects of care associated with urinary tract infection (UTI) is determining the criteria that define it. In the past, a urinary bacterial count of greater than 100,000/mL was sufficient to make a diagnosis of infection, and diagnosis would be followed by antibiotic treatment. More recently, however, geriatricians have questioned both this criterion for infection and the use of antibiotics in individuals who are otherwise asymptomatic. That is, asymptomatic bacteriuria is not an infection and should not be treated.

Nursing home residents, especially the elderly, have a tendency to establish multiple bacterial colonies in their urine. Therefore, routine urine cultures are clinically useless and costly. If the bacteria or other pathogen invade the bladder wall and cause clinical manifestations, *then* the resident needs treatment. The risk of antibiotic therapy in an elderly person far outweighs the risk that the individual might develop an infection from the bacteriuria.

Women are more at risk for UTIs than men because women have shorter urethras that are in close proximity to the vagina and rectum (sources of bacteria). One of the most common causative organisms for UTIs is *Escherichia coli*, found in feces. Other causative pathogens include *Enterococcus*, *Klebsiella*, *Proteus*, and *Pseudomonas* bacteria (Ignatavicius, Workman, & Mishler, 1995). If not treated, a UTI can lead to septicemia, a generalized infection caused by urosepsis. Urosepsis leads a high mortality rate in the elderly.

Prevention

One of the most important preventive measures for UTIs is to monitor those residents who are most at risk for developing them. High risk residents include:

- The elderly, especially those who are diabetic or have neuromuscular conditions (e.g., stroke) that cause urinary retention
- Those on long-term steroid therapy (steroids depress the immune system)
- Those who are immunocompromised (e.g., by HIV infection)
- Those who have urinary retention from obstructive causes, such as benign prostatic hypertrophy.

Urinary tract infection resulting from long-term urinary catheter use has declined because catheters are not used as often as they were in the past. The longer the catheter stays in place, the more likely the individual is to get an infection. Residents who have been catheterized for more than 30 days usually colonize bacteria but may be asymptomatic. Daily catheter care may decrease the incidence of UTI in catheterized residents.

Other strategies for preventing UTIs include increasing fluid intake for all residents, unless otherwise contraindicated, and toileting residents on a regular schedule to prevent urinary retention. When urine remains in the bladder, it is more likely to be colonized by bacteria.

Assessment

The classic signs and symptoms of a urinary tract infection are urinary frequency, urgency, and dysuria (painful urination). The urine is typically cloudy, darker than usual, and has a foul odor. However, an elderly resident may present with more vague clinical manifestations, such as confusion, restlessness, or other atypical behavior. A positive culture and sensitivity along with these manifestations confirms a diagnosis of infection.

Interventions

If the resident has an obstructive problem, such as prostatic hypertrophy, the obstruction needs to be relieved to prevent urinary retention. The physician or other health care provider also prescribes the appropriate antibiotic therapy. Adequate hydration to help flush the urinary tract is important, as well as monitoring both amount and characteristics of the resident's urine.

The nurse teaches the resident, family, and direct care staff about the need for toileting and proper hygiene. After toileting, the female perineal area should be cleansed from the front (the mons pubis) to the back (anal area). This helps prevent contamination of the urinary meatus by fecal material.

Fluid Imbalances

In the average adult, fluid (primarily water) constitutes 60 percent of the body weight. In the elderly, this figure is less than 50 percent. Women typically have less body fluid than men (Lee, Barrett, & Ignatavicius, 1996). Therefore, elderly women are at the highest risk for emergencies related to fluid imbalances.

The two major imbalances are fluid volume deficit and fluid volume overload. Electrolyte imbalances usually accompany these imbalances.

Although many fluid and electrolyte imbalances can occur in nursing home residents for a number of reasons, only the most common ones are presented here.

FLUID VOLUME DEFICIT

Fluid volume deficit, most commonly referred to as dehydration, is a very common problem among nursing home residents, particularly the elderly. Dehydration may be an *actual* decrease in body fluid, due to fluid losses or inadequate fluid intake; or a *relative* decrease, in which fluid (plasma) leaves the intravascular compartment (bloodstream) and goes into the interstitial spaces, a process known as "third spacing."

Definition

The elderly resident usually experiences an actual loss of body fluid. Many factors place the elderly at risk for dehydration, such as decreased fluid intake, fever, infection, diuresis, decreased fluid intake, bleeding, vomiting, and diarrhea. Physiologic changes associated with aging inhibit compensatory mechanisms that can help maintain fluid balance. For example, declining kidney function prevents the conservation of water and sodium in the body. In addition, the elderly have a high risk of developing illnesses that cause fluid imbalances, such as urinary tract infection and diabetes mellitus (see later discussion of hyperglycemia, hyperosmolar nonketotic syndrome). Diuretics are commonly used for the elderly and can cause dehydration and electrolyte imbalances if the resident is not carefully monitored.

Prevention

The best way to prevent fluid deficit in nursing home residents is to keep them well hydrated and monitor residents who are at the highest risk for dehydration. The elderly have a diminished thirst response and, therefore, usually need encouragement to drink fluids. Ensuring adequate fluid intake is better managed by providing the resident with frequent sips of favorite beverages rather than expecting the resident to drink an entire glass of fluid.

Monitoring laboratory values of serum electrolytes, especially sodium, blood urea nitrogen (BUN), and hematocrit is another important preventive strategy. Depending on the cause of the fluid deficit, the sodium levels may decrease, increase, or remain within normal limits. The BUN typically increases in residents with dehydration because the kidneys attempt to conserve body water to compensate for fluid loss. The hematocrit usually increases because it represents the percentage of red blood cells to the plasma. As the plasma decreases, the percentage of cells to fluid increases, a condition known as hemoconcentration.

Assessment

In addition to laboratory assessment, the nurse relies on physical assessment findings. Because the resident experiencing dehydration is hypovolemic, the cardiovascular and renal systems are affected. Typical assessment findings are listed in Table 6–2.

Interventions

The goals of management are to restore fluid and electrolytes as needed and to treat the cause of dehydration. For mild dehydration, oral fluid replacement is usually sufficient. For more severe dehydration, intravenous fluid replacement may be needed as well.

Oral rehydration therapy (ORT) has been successfully used in the nursing home setting as an option for replacing both fluid and electrolyte losses caused by severe diarrhea. ORT is more cost-effective than intravenous therapy and is particularly useful for residents who have adequate renal and cardiovascular function. Table 6–3 lists examples of ORT solutions and their composition.

The nurse also provides comfort measures for dry skin and mucous membranes, such as body lotion and oral care. The staff assists the resident when changing position to prevent falls, which can result from postural hypotension.

FLUID VOLUME OVERLOAD

Fluid volume overload usually results from an actual excess of water in the body, either from excessive fluid intake or inadequate fluid excretion by the kidneys.

Table 6–2. **Typical Physical Assessment Findings Associated with Fluid Volume Deficit (Dehydration)**

- Decreased blood pressure
- Postural hypotension (systolic pressure decreased by more than 20 mmHg when the resident changes from a supine to a sitting or standing position)
- Increased pulse rate
- Increased temperature
- Decreased urinary output
- Dark, concentrated urine
- Weight loss (the best indicator of fluid loss)
- Dry, warm skin; dry, sticky mucous membranes
- Poor skin turgor (test the skin over the sternum or forehead for the most accurate results)
- Confusion and disorientation
- Soft, sunken eyeballs

Table 6–3 **Commercial Solutions for Oral Rehydration Therapy**

Brand Name	Na$^+$ (mEq/L)	K$^+$ (mEq/L)	Cl$^-$ (mEq/L)	Citrate (mEq/L)	Sugar or Starch	Calories (kcal) per Liter
Ricelyte (Mead-Johnson)	50	25	45	34	Rice syrup 30 g)	126
Resol (Wyeth-Ayerst)	50	20	50	34	Dextrose (20 g)	84
Rehydralyte (Ross Labs)	75	20	65	30	Dextrose (25 g)	100
Pedialyte (Ross Labs)	45	20	35	30	Dextrose (25 g)	100
Gastrolyte (Rorer)	60	20	60	10	Dextrose (17.8 g)	75
Rapolyte (Richmond)	90	20	80	30	Dextrose (20 g)	84

Definition

Like dehydration, fluid overload occurring in the elderly resident is usually due to the inability of the kidneys to compensate for fluid excess. In the nursing home resident, the major cause of fluid overload is heart failure. Physiologic changes associated with aging, such as myocardial hypertrophy, coronary artery arteriosclerosis, and decreased circulation, contribute to the failure of the heart as a pump. The heart is unable to pump effectively and blood (fluid) backs up into the heart, lungs (left congestive heart failure [CHF]), and systemic circulation (right CHF).

Prevention

In many cases, congestive heart failure cannot be prevented. If the individual's heart is diseased or injured from previous myocardial infarctions or other cardiac problem, CHF is likely to occur. As with other acute illnesses and health emergencies, part of illness prevention is to identify those residents who are most at risk. Risk factors for heart failure include:

- Age over 65 years
- A history of heart disease and hypertension
- A history of renal disease
- A history of chronic lung disease
- One or more previous episodes of congestive heart failure

For individuals at high risk, fluid consumption may need to be restricted and the resident may require a regimen of diuretics to facilitate excess fluid excretion. A sodium-restricted diet is also helpful because sodium causes fluid retention, which must be avoided. Intravenous therapy must be closely monitored to prevent fluid overload and extra work for the heart.

Assessment

Clinical findings from the physical assessment are more useful than laboratory testing when assessing the resident experiencing fluid overload. The primary clinical manifestations involve the cardiovascular and respiratory systems, as listed in Table 6–4.

Interventions

The resident with fluid overload related to congestive heart failure typically experiences dyspnea. The priority intervention is to raise the head of the bed and administer oxygen at a low concentration (2–3 L/min). The health care provider orders a diuretic, usually furosemide (Lasix) or bumetanide (Bumex) to be given either orally (mild failure) or intravenously (more serious failure). Angiotensin converting enzyme (ACE)

Table 6–4. **Physical Assessment Findings in Residents with Fluid Overload**

Increased pulse rate
Bounding pulses
Increased blood pressure
Distended neck and hand veins
Increased respiratory rate
Shallow, labored respirations
Crackles
Dependent edema
Disorientation or confusion
Pale, clammy skin
Restlessness

---

inhibitors, such as lisinopril (Zestril) and quinapril (Accupril), are given to residents with heart failure to increase cardiac output and decrease peripheral vascular resistance (afterload).

Early detection of CHF is crucial to prevent a life-threatening complication called pulmonary edema. In pulmonary edema, the lungs become filled with fluid; mortality rates are very high. The resident must be hospitalized and may be placed on a ventilator during the acute phase.

Common Electrolyte Imbalances

In the body, serum electrolytes must be maintained in a delicate balance to promote the optimal function of cells. However, a number of conditions and medications can lead to imbalances, many of which can be life-threatening. Two acute imbalances, hypokalemia (decreased serum potassium) and hyponatremia (decreased serum sodium), are common among nursing home residents.

DEFINITIONS

Hypokalemia occurs when the serum potassium falls below 3.5 mEq/L. It may be caused by a decreased intake of potassium or, more likely, by an excessive loss of potassium from the body. The most common cause of hypokalemia is the overuse or prolonged use of non-potassium-sparing diuretics, such as loop (high-ceiling) and thiazide diuretics. Furosemide (Lasix) and bumetanide (Bumex) are typically used loop diuretics; metolazone (Zaroxolyn) and indapamide (Lozol) are typically used thiazides.

Diuretics work by increasing the excretion of sodium and water (water follows sodium). Therefore, diuretics are also a major cause of sodium deficit. *Hyponatremia* occurs when the serum sodium falls below 135 mEq/L.

The second major reason for potassium loss is vomiting and diarrhea. Gastrointestinal (GI) contents are rich in sodium and potassium, and losses from the GI tract cause hypokalemia and hyponatremia.

PREVENTION

Electrolyte imbalances can be prevented by carefully monitoring laboratory results and identifying high-risk residents. The elderly resident and other residents with hypertension and heart disease are most likely to be administered diuretics as part of their treatment plan. For these residents, eating foods high in potassium, such as bananas, melons, and citrus fruits, may help prevent a deficit. For some residents, an oral potassium supplement may be taken daily.

Although many residents taking diuretics need a sodium-restricted diet, caution must be taken to provide enough sodium to meet the body's needs. Hyponatremia is sometimes referred to as a "silent killer" because the individual often has no clinical manifestations and is undiagnosed.

ASSESSMENT

Potassium is needed for the function of cardiac, skeletal, and smooth muscle in the body. When it is decreased, these muscles do not function properly, causing weakness, decreased GI motility, and dysrhythmias.

Sodium is needed for all cells, especially those of the central nervous system. When sodium decreases, the resident's level of consciousness and mental state declines, causing disorientation, confusion, and lethargy. If the resident is not treated, the condition may progress to coma and death.

Assessment of clinical manifestations alone is not sufficient in monitoring for potassium and sodium imbalances. Frequent electrolyte studies, at least monthly, must be drawn for residents who are at high risk for these potentially life-threatening problems.

INTERVENTIONS

Once the deficit has been identified, replacement of the electrolytes and correcting the cause of the imbalance become the goals of treatment. In severe deficits, the resident may require hospitalization and intravenous replacement.

Diabetic Emergencies

Diabetes mellitus is a chronic disease in which inadequate production or utilization of insulin results in increased blood sugar. It is is very common, especially in the elderly population. Diabetes is classified into two types—type I and type II. Type I diabetics are insulin dependent and are typically children or young adults. Most diabetics, though, have type II diabetes and are not insulin dependent. Their blood sugar is controlled by diet, oral hypoglycemic agents, or both. Type II diabetics tend to be middle-aged and older adults.

Complications from diabetes can affect every body system. Some complications are chronic, such as peripheral neuropathy, retinopathy, or renal failure, and take years to develop.

Other complications are acute and can develop in a matter of hours. Acute complications, including hypoglycemia and hyperglycemia, can become life-threatening emergencies if not prevented or detected early.

HYPOGLYCEMIA

Hypoglycemia is an acute complication of diabetes mellitus in which the blood sugar becomes too low to meet the needs of the body. Both type I and type II diabetics can experience this problem.

Definition

Hypoglycemia occurs when the resident's blood sugar (serum glucose) falls below 70 mg/dL. The cells of the brain and other body cells need glucose for fuel to function adequately. When they are deprived of this fuel for a prolonged period of time, death can result.

Prevention

Hypoglycemia usually occurs when there is not enough food (sugar) intake to balance the insulin in the body. Therefore, prevention focuses on following a treatment plan that keeps the blood sugar within normal limits (70–110 mg/dL). If the resident takes insulin or oral agents that stimulate insulin production but fails to eat, the blood sugar drops.

As the blood sugar begins to decline, the resident feels lightheaded, disoriented, or fatigued. Providing a quick source of sugar to the resident usually reverses the symptoms and prevents a life-threatening situation. Fast-acting sources of sugar include hard candy, unsweetened orange juice, milk, honey, graham crackers, and peanut butter.

The nurse teaches the resident and family the signs and symptoms of hypoglycemia so that they can be reported promptly. An available source of sugar should be readily accessible for the resident to use when needed.

Assessment

The early manifestations of hypoglycemia result from lack of glucose to the brain. The resident becomes disoriented and confused (or more confused than usual), and may be lightheaded or dizzy. The skin is cool, sweaty, and clammy, and the resident may feel shaky and hungry. If the situation is not assessed and acted upon quickly, the resident can progress rapidly into a coma and die.

Although finger stick blood sugar (FSBS) devices are available, they should not replace the nurse's clinical judgment. If the resident seems to be having a hypoglycemic reaction, the nurse needs to act accordingly.

Interventions

The primary intervention for hypoglycemia is glucose replacement. If the resident is unconscious (severe hypoglycemia) and therefore cannot consume anything by mouth, 50 percent IV dextrose or subcutaneous glucagon must be used. These should be on hand for such emergencies. A second dose may be given if the resident remains unconscious (Ignatavicius et al., 1995).

HYPERGLYCEMIA

Hyperglycemia is an acute complication of diabetes mellitus in which the blood sugar becomes too high. Two hyperglycemic complications may occur—diabetic ketoacidosis and hyperglycemic, hyperosmolar nonketotic syndrome (Table 6–5).

Definitions

Diabetic ketoacidosis (DKA) occurs in individuals who have type I diabetes. In this complication, the body is unable to produce enough insulin to move the glucose into the cells for fuel and, therefore, breaks down fatty acids for fuel. The end products of this fat metabolism are called ketones or ketone bodies.

Hyperglycemic, hyperosmolar nonketotic syndrome (HHNKS), sometimes referred to as the hyperosmolar syndrome, occurs in individuals

Table 6–5. **Physical Findings in Hyperglycemic Emergencies**

Diabetic Ketoacidosis	Hyperglycemic, Hyperosmolar Nonketotic Syndrome
Blood glucose over 300 mg/dL	Blood glucose over 600 mg/dL
Signs and symptoms of dehydration	Signs and symptoms of severe dehydration
Metabolic acidosis	No acidosis
Kussmaul's respiration	No changes in breathing
Fruity, sweet breath	No changes in breath odor
Warm, dry skin	Warm, dry skin
Fatigue	Fatigue

who have type II diabetes. In this complication, even though the body is unable to produce enough insulin to move glucose into the cells, fatty acids are *not* broken down and no ketosis is present. As the blood glucose continues to increase, the resident with HHNKS can become comatose, a condition known as hyperglycemic, hyperosmolar nonketotic coma (HHNKC).

Prevention

Like the preventive measures for hypoglycemia, prevention for hyperglycemic reactions focuses on balancing the body's sugar intake with its available insulin. If the resident does not follow the diabetic diet and consumes too much sugar, hyperglycemia results. Health teaching is a crucial preventive measure.

Because DKA and HHNKS are often precipitated by infection or other acute illness, preventing infection is another important health promotion strategy. Proper handwashing, special foot care, adequate hydration, and avoiding others who have infections are some of the ways that a diabetic can prevent infection.

Concurrent acute health problems, such as myocardial infarction, pancreatitis, and stroke, can cause HHNKS. Certain drugs, such as glucocorticoids (prednisone), beta-adrenergic blocking agents, calcium channel blockers, and phenytoin sodium (Dilantin) can also lead to HHNKS.

Assessment

As for all acute illnesses or emergencies, the health care team must identify those residents who are at high risk for hyperglycemic complications and monitor their blood glucose levels carefully. When a diabetic resident becomes acutely ill, the balance of sugar and insulin is affected and an acute diabetic complication is likely to occur.

Although both DKA and HHNKS are hyperglycemia complications, the clinical manifestations and diagnostic assessment of each condition are somewhat different. Early detection of these complications is crucial because mortality rates, especially for HHNKS, are very high among the elderly.

The onset for *DKA* is usually very sudden. The resident typically has a serum glucose greater than 300 mg/dL and has polyuria (excessive urination to eliminate the increased glucose) and polydipsia (excessive thirst). Dehydration and sodium loss are common, along with weight loss; dry, warm skin; lethargy; and sunken, soft eyeballs. Ketosis causes metabolic acidosis and hyperkalemia (increased serum potassium). The body attempts to compensate for the increased acid state by "blowing off" extra carbon dioxide by the lungs. The resident's respiratory pattern is therefore typically rapid and deep (Kussmaul's respiration) and the breath has a fruity, sweet smell. Nausea and abdominal pain may also be present.

The onset of *HHNKS* is more gradual, developing slowly over days or weeks. The serum glucose is usually over 800 mg/dL, but clinical manifestations may begin at 600 mg/dL. Because the resident with HHNKS has no ketosis, metabolic acidosis and Kussmaul's respirations do *not* occur. However, dehydration with electrolyte loss (as described earlier) is very common and causes central nervous system changes, including confusion, lethargy, and eventually coma if the resident is not treated. Renal impairment usually results because blood flow to the kidneys decreases as the blood becomes more hyperosmolar (more concentrated).

Interventions

Interventions for both hyperglycemic emergencies include treatment of the underlying cause, such as infection, and the administration of fluids and regular insulin. Intravenous fluids are needed to correct the fluid and electrolyte imbalances. Intravenous insulin is used to bring the serum glucose level within normal range.

Myocardial Infarction

Myocardial infarction (MI), also known as a "heart attack," is the result of coronary artery disease (CAD), a common problem among nursing home residents. CAD is the leading cause of death in the United States. It affects the small arteries that supply oxygen and nutrients to the myocardium (heart muscle), resulting in ischemia and sometimes necrosis of myocardial cells (infarction).

DEFINITION

Arteriosclerosis (loss of arterial wall elasticity) and atherosclerosis (fatty, fibrous plaques on the arterial walls) are the major contributors to CAD. The lumens of the coronary arteries narrow, thus restricting blood flow to the heart muscle. The myocardium requires a large amount of oxygen. When deprived of oxygen, ischemia occurs and causes chest pain *(angina)*. If the resident experiences angina, the warning sign of CAD, the ischemia is limited in duration and causes no permanent myocardial damage or tissue necrosis.

An MI occurs when the heart muscle is abruptly and severely deprived of oxygen, causing long-term ischemia and tissue injury. The damaged muscle releases cardiac enzymes (creatine kinase [CK] and lactate dehydrogenase [LDH]) into the bloodstream. These can be measured by laboratory assessment. The values are elevated in the resident with an MI but not in the resident experiencing angina.

PREVENTION

Research has shown that a number of risk factors contribute to the incidence of CAD. Some of these factors cannot be modified or controlled, such as being over 65 years of age or having a family history of heart disease. The risk of CAD can be reduced by minimizing or avoiding controllable risk factors, such as smoking, obesity, hypertension, elevated serum cholesterol, physical inactivity, and high stress levels.

In the nursing home setting, the health team can work together to plan care that minimizes some of the risk factors, by providing a low-cholesterol and/or low-fat diet, control of hypertension, and increased physical activity for the resident. Resident education regarding risk factors may also help to reduce the risk of MIs (see Chapter 8). Some elderly residents feel that they have lived long enough to engage in any lifestyle they wish, which includes smoking and eating whatever they want. The health team must respect the resident's lifestyle and quality of life, and allow the resident to make decisions about his or her health.

ASSESSMENT AND INTERVENTIONS

The nurse needs to be aware that the manifestations of angina and myocardial infarction are similar, but the results are not (Table 6–6). Angina causes chest pain and anxiety, and is precipitated by activity or other stressor. Rest or nitroglycerin (NTG, a sublingual coronary vasodilator) usually relieves anginal pain. Up to three NTG tablets given 5 minutes

Table 6–6. **Classic Key Features of Angina and Myocardial Infarction**

Angina	Myocardial Infarction
Substernal chest discomfort	Substernal chest pressure
▪ Radiating to the left arm	▪ Radiating to the left arm, back, or jaw
▪ Precipitated by exertion or stress	▪ Occurring without cause, primarily early in the morning
▪ Relieved by nitroglycerin or rest	▪ Relieved only by opioids
▪ Lasting <15 min.	▪ Lasting 30 min or more
▪ Few associated symptoms	▪ Frequent associated symptoms:
	▫ Nausea
	▫ Diaphoresis
	▫ Dyspnea
	▫ Feelings of fear and anxiety
	▫ Dysrhythmias

From *Medical-Surgical Nursing: A Nursing Process Approach* (p. 990), by D. D. Ignatavicius, M. L. Workman, and M. A. Mishler, 1995, Philadelphia: W. B. Saunders. Reprinted with permission.

apart may be used. If no pain relief is achieved after three tablets or rest, the resident must be transported to the hospital immediately by a life support team.

A resident experiencing an MI may or may not have the classic signs and symptoms of crushing chest pain, anxiety, diaphoresis, and nausea. Many elderly residents complain only of indigestion or have jaw pain. They may become disoriented or confused. These vague manifestations may be overlooked until the resident experiences cardiogenic shock, a severe form of heart failure resulting from the infarction.

Vascular Emergencies

Because many nursing home residents are elderly and have physiologic changes in their cardiovascular systems, vascular emergencies are fairly common. Examples of vascular emergencies include cerebrovascular accident (CVA) and peripheral vascular occlusion—deep vein thrombosis and acute arterial occlusion.

CEREBROVASCULAR ACCIDENT

Cerebrovascular accident, or "stroke," is a common problem among middle-aged and older adults. The risk factors for CVA are similar to those described in the previous section for myocardial infarction. The elderly, especially those with uncontrolled hypertension, are most at risk.

Definition

A CVA is an ischemic process that affects the nerve cells of the brain. The resident experiences a CVA when, in a scenario resembling myocardial infarctions, the cells of the brain are deprived of oxygen due to narrowing or occlusion (thrombosis) of cerebral or extracranial (such as the carotid) arteries. The resident may recover fully without permanent dysfunction or may have neurologic impairments that interfere with the ability to perform activities of daily living or to communicate.

Prevention

Some residents experience transient ischemic attacks (TIAs), lasting less than 24 hours, in which a temporary neurologic deficit occurs. Residents who experience TIAs have narrowing of cerebral or carotid arteries and may be placed on maintenance anticoagulation with low-dose aspirin or another agent to prevent additional accumulation of the causative plaque (clot).

Other preventive strategies are similar to those described in the previous section on MI. Reducing modifiable risk factors may minimize the risk of a CVA. Controlling hypertension through diet and/or medication is probably one of the most important preventive measures. Severe hypertension can cause small cerebral vessels to rupture, a process known as hemorrhagic stroke.

Assessment

The physical findings associated with a CVA depend on the location of the ischemia in the brain. Most strokes involve the middle cerebral artery, which supplies the areas of the brain controlling voluntary movement, sensation, speech, language, memory, perception, and judgment. Because each side of the brain functions somewhat independently, only one side of the brain is affected. A left-sided stroke causes symptoms on the right side of the body and vice versa because the nerve fibers cross at the medulla before descending into the spinal cord and into the periphery. Table 6–7 summarizes the typical physical assessment findings associated with left- and right-sided CVAs.

Table 6–7. **Key Features of Left and Right Hemisphere Cerebrovascular Accidents**

Feature	Left Hemisphere*	Right Hemisphere
Language	• Aphasia • Agraphia • Alexia	• Impaired sense of humor
Memory	• Deficit may be present	• Disoriented to time, place, and person • Cannot recognize faces
Vision	• Unable to discriminate words and letters • Reading problems • Deficits in the right visual field	• Visual spatial deficits • Neglect of the left visual field • Loss of depth perception
Behavior	• Slow • Cautious • Anxious when attempting a new task • Depression or a catastrophic response to illness • Sense of guilt • Feeling of worthlessness • Worries over future • Quick anger and frustration	• Impulsive • Unaware of neurologic deficits • Confabulates • Euphoric • Constantly smiles • Denies illness • Poor judgment • Overestimates abilities (risk for injury)
Hearing	• No deficit	• Loses ability to hear tonal variations

*Location for speech in all but 15% to 20% of people.
From *Medical-Surgical Nursing: A Nursing Process Approach* (p. 1251), by D. D. Ignatavicius, M. L. Workman, and M. A. Mishler, 1995, Philadelphia: W. B. Saunders. Reprinted with permission.

Interventions

The most important initial intervention is to assess the resident for early signs and symptoms of increasing intracranial pressure, such as decreased level of consciousness. Placing the resident in a sitting position helps to decrease intracranial pressure. A complete neurologic assessment is performed to determine functional impairments. A resident with a mild stroke may remain in the facility, but residents with more severe strokes are sent to the hospital for evaluation and stabilization.

The resident returns to the nursing home for continuation of an aggressive rehabilitation program.

ACUTE PERIPHERAL VASCULAR OCCLUSION

Many nursing home residents have chronic peripheral vascular disease. These residents tend to be over 70 years of age, have diabetes mellitus, and have decreased mobility.

Acute peripheral vascular problems, including deep vein thrombosis (DVT) and acute arterial occlusion, can affect people of any age. DVT is more common, but arterial occlusion may be more life-threatening.

Definitions

As the name implies, *deep vein thrombosis* is the formation of a clot in a deep vein, usually of the calf or thigh. As the clot slows the return of the venous blood to the heart, the blood clot increases in size and obstructs peripheral venous flow. The major complication of a DVT is an embolus in which a part of the clot breaks away and circulates through the body. The embolus may then lodge in the lung, causing pulmonary embolism; the brain, causing a CVA; or the heart, causing an MI. All of these thromboembolitic conditions are life-threatening.

Arterial occlusion involves the same process as deep vein thrombosis but occurs in an artery, often the femoral or pelvic artery. Decreased arterial blood flow contributes to clot formation. The major complication of an arterial clot is irreversible tissue damage to the leg, which may necessitate distal amputation.

Prevention

Prevention of acute peripheral vascular occlusion includes increased mobility, leg exercises, anti-embolitic stockings, adequate hydration, and anticoagulant therapy. The individual most at risk for DVT is the elderly resident who has had hip surgery. These preventive measures are used for up to 2 months postoperatively to reduce the risk of thromboembolitic complications.

Other high-risk residents are those who have been immobilized for a prolonged period of time and those who have a history of acute or chronic vascular problems.

Assessment

Although both types of acute occlusions usually affect the lower extremi ties, the physical assessment findings are quite different. For example, the skin over the site of DVT is warm and swollen. The skin of the resident with an arterial occlusion is cold and clammy below the occlusion site. The distal pulses are either absent or decreased. Pain is common in both conditions. The pain associated with DVT tends to be localized, however, while the pain from an acute arterial occlusion is diffuse, affecting the entire leg. Table 6–8 differentiates the common clinical manifestations associated with these vascular problems.

Interventions

The most important intervention is early detection and management. Intravenous heparin is the initial drug of choice to prevent growth of the existing clot and the development of further clots. The resident needs to be immobilized until the clot begins to resolve to prevent emboli. Adequate hydration is also important. On return to the nursing home, the resident will continue with an oral anticoagulant. The nursing staff should observe for signs of bleeding or excessive bruising.

Coagulation values are carefully monitored to ensure that the resident is receiving a therapeutic amount of medication but not so much as to cause bleeding. The prothrombin time (PT) or International Normalized Ratio (INR) are used to monitor residents on warfarin (Coumadin). The partial thromboplastin time (PTT) or activated partial thromboplastin time (APTT) are used to monitor residents on heparin.

Table 6–8. **Common Clinical Manifestations of Deep Vein Thrombosis and Acute Arterial Occlusion**

Deep Vein Thrombosis	Acute Arterial Occlusion
Primarily affects lower extremities	Primarily affects lower extremities
Pain is localized near clot	Pain is diffuse and severe
Skin warm and affected area swollen	Extremity cool or cold
Area reddened	Leg pale, mottled, or cyanotic
Pulses not usually affected	Decreased or absent distal pulses
	Decreased capillary refills
	Venous congestion
	Tender, indurated muscles

Drugs that counteract anticoagulants should be available in the emergency drug box. Vitamin K is the antidote for warfarin; protamine sulfate is the antidote for heparin.

CHAPTER HIGHLIGHTS

The two major respiratory infections that affect nursing home residents are influenza and pneumonia.

Influenza and pneumonia vaccines reduce the risk of respiratory infection among nursing home residents.

Pneumonia and urosepsis have high mortality rates in the elderly.

The elderly are at high risk for both fluid volume deficit (dehydration) and fluid volume overload.

The major cause of fluid overload among nursing home residents is congestive heart failure.

Hypokalemia and hyponatremia are common electrolyte imbalances experienced by nursing home residents.

The three diabetic emergencies are hypoglycemia, diabetic ketoacidosis (DKA), and hyperglycemic, hyperosmolar nonketotic syndrome (HHNKS).

DKA, occurring in type I diabetics, and HHNKS, occurring in type II diabetics, are both characterized by hyperglycemia and dehydration.

A cerebrovascular accident occurs when blood flow to a part of the brain is diminished, resulting in neurologic dysfunction.

Deep vein thrombosis (DVT) and acute arterial occlusion typically affect the lower extremities.

The primary concern with DVT is the risk of embolism to major body organs.

REFERENCES AND READINGS

Centers for Disease Control and Prevention. (1995). Pneumonia and influenza rates—United States 1979–1994. *MMWR, 44*, 535–537.

Cunha, B. A., Gingrich, D., & Rosebaum, G. S. (1990). Pneumonia syndromes: A clinical approach in the elderly. *Geriatrics, 45*, 49–55.

Fein, A. M., Feinsilver, S. H., & Niederman, M. S. (1991). The elusive diagnosis of pneumonia in the elderly. *Emergency Medicine, 23*, 87–96.

Ignatavicius, D. D., Workman, M. L., & Mishler, M. (1995). *Medical-surgical nursing: A nursing process approach*. Philadelphia: W. B. Saunders.

Lee, C. A., Barrett, A., & Ignatavicius, D. D. (1996). *Fluids and electrolytes: A practical approach*. Philadelphia: F. A. Davis.

Long, C. O., Isemeurt, R., & Wilson, L. W. (1995). The elderly and pneumonia: Prevention and management. *Home Health Care Nurse, 13*(5), 43–47.

Matteson, M. A., McConnell, E. S., & Linton, A. D. (1997). *Gerontological nursing: Concepts and practice*. Philadelphia: W. B. Saunders.

DISCUSSION QUESTIONS TO PROMOTE CRITICAL THINKING

1. A nursing assistant reports that one of your residents seems more tired than usual today. Her blood pressure is low and her pulse is unusually high. The resident is a type II diabetic with a history of congestive heart failure. She is taking Lasix and a KCl supplement. What additional assessment data should you collect at this time?

2. In the scenario described in the previous question, for what fluid and/or electrolyte imbalance(s) is the resident at risk?

3. As a type II diabetic, what emergent condition is she likely to develop?

4. One of your residents tells you that her right leg is throbbing. On assessment you find that the leg is cool, mottled, and painful. Her right pedal and posterior tibial pulses are weaker than her left pulses. What problem should you suspect that she is experiencing and what action should you take?

7 Documentation Requirements in the Nursing Home

OUTLINE

Comprehensive Resident Care Plan
Clinical Pathway
Progress Notes
Skin Assessment Record
Medication Administration Record
Activity and Treatment Record
Incident Report

OBJECTIVES

- Identify the difference between a traditional comprehensive resident care plan and a clinical pathway
- List four purposes of documenting resident progress
- Describe three methods for charting resident progress
- Identify the purposes of the skin assessment record, medication administration record, activity and treatment record, and incident report

Compared to that in other health care settings, documentation in nursing homes is very complex and time-consuming. Chapter 3 described the admission assessment form, the Minimum Data Set (MDS), and the Resident Assessment Protocols (RAPS) that are required for every resident. (See also Appendix C.)

Based on the assessment findings from these documents, a comprehensive, interdisciplinary resident care plan is developed and updated as needed or required by regulation. In addition to the care plan, nurses use a number of other chart forms to document resident progress. Although specific chart forms may vary depending on facility policy, the following discussion outlines the basic purpose and principles of the most commonly used parts of the medical record in a nursing home.

Comprehensive Resident Care Plan

State and federal laws mandate that every resident in a nursing home must have an interdisciplinary resident care plan. Members of the health care team meet as needed, usually at least once a week, to initiate, review, or update the care plan. Some of the residents' problems on the plan are triggered by the MDS. Other problems, such as additional nursing diagnoses, can be added as appropriate (see Appendix D).

The care plan lists one or more expected outcomes for each resident problem. Then the interventions that help the resident meet the outcomes are specified. The evaluation column is used to describe the achievement of outcomes and revision of the plan, if any.

Each care plan must be reviewed, evaluated, and updated at least every 90 days on a traditional nursing home unit. Residents who qualify for Medicare for skilled care must have 30-day reviews. Residents receiving medical assistance funding may require 60- or 90-day reviews, depending on state policy. If the resident's condition changes significantly at any time, a new MDS and care plan must be documented within 14 days of the change.

Clinical Pathway

The clinical pathway (CP) is the newest method for developing a plan of care for a resident. Sometimes called a care map, critical path, or collaborative plan of care, the CP is an interdisciplinary guideline for care that outlines expected outcomes and the sequence of interventions across a time line. The sample pathway in Figure 7–1 shows the care provided from preadmission, through the hospital stay, and into the nursing home or home. This pathway could be extended to outline the care provided in

Clinical Pathway for Total Hip Replacement

ICD-9 Code 715.35

Nursing Diagnosis/Collaborative Problem	Expected Outcome (The Patient Is Expected to...)	Met/Not Met	Reason
Pain	State that pain is relieved following appropriate interventions		
Potential for dislocation	Not experience dislocation of the operative hip		
Potential for postoperative complications (hemorrhage, infection, thromboembolitic complications)	Have Hgb and Hct WNL, stable VS, WBC WNL, and no S/S of DVT, PE, or other thromboembolitic complications		
Impaired physical mobility	Walk from room into hall using a walker with supervision; not experience complications of immobility		

Aspect of Care	Date ___ Pre-admission/Pre-op	Date ___ Day 1 (DOS)	Date ___ Day 2 (POD #1)	Date ___ Day 3 (POD #2)	Date ___ Day 4 (POD #3)	Date ___ Day 5 (POD #4)
Assessment	Systems assessment Pre-op checklist Psychosocial assessment PT evaluation for assistive/ambulatory aids; muscle strength (UE and LE)	PACU: Systems assessment Pain assessment VS q 15 min x 4, q 30 min x 4 NV checks with VS Check hip dressing and drain	VS and NV assessment q 4 h; check hip dressing and drain Maintain hip abduction; keep operative leg in alignment (may use knee immobilizer)	VS q 8 h with NV checks Assess for BM Assess incision for S/S of infection Maintain hip abduction/assess for dislocation Assess skin q 8 h	VS q 8 h with NV checks Assess hip incision for S/S of infection Assess LE for S/S of DVT Assess for results of laxative, if given	Same as Day 4 (POD #3)

Maintain hip abduction with pillow or special device (assess position) *Post-op:* Pain assessment VS q 1 h x 4, then q 4 h with NV checks Monitor hip dressing for drainage and drain function Systems assessment Check for voiding Assess skin (especially heels) q 8 h	Assess skin (especially heels) q 8 h Nutritional assessment, if needed Systems assessment q 8–12 h	Same as Day 2 (POD #1)	Assess skin, especially heels QD	Review discharge instruction
Teaching Pre-op teaching regarding surgery; pain management, post-op expectations, hip precautions PT instruction regarding use of walker and weight-bearing expected post-op Review plan of care/clinical pathway with patient and family	Teach/demonstrate DB & C techniques; incentive spirometer Reinforce basic understanding of surgical procedure Hip precautions Teach/demonstrate procedure for ankle pumps, quad and gluteal sets	Reinforce teaching regarding hip precautions Reinforce teaching regarding LE exercises Teach additional pain relief measures, such as muscle relaxation and visual imagery, if appropriate Teach purpose of anticoagulation measures	Begin discharge teaching regarding • Wound care • Pain management • Physical activity/ sexual activity • Ambulation/ weight-bearing exercises • Rehabilitation program complications • Meds • Hip precautions • Bleeding precautions/testing	

Figure 7-1. Sample clinical pathway.

Clinical Pathway for Total Hip Replacement Continued

Aspect of Care (Cont'd)	Date _____ Pre-admission/ Pre-op	Date _____ Day 1 (DOS)	Date _____ Day 2 (POD #1)	Date _____ Day 3 (POD #2)	Date _____ Day 4 (POD #3)	Date _____ Day 5 (POD #4)
Consults	PT for evaluation	Social worker for rehab/placement	PT for muscle strengthening exercises and post-op evaluation	PT for weight-bearing and ambulation with walker	N/A	N/A
Lab Tests	Admission labs, including CBC, SMA-6 (6/60), INR(PT)/APTT	N/A	Hgb and Hct (contact MD if Hgb ≤9 or Hct ≤28)(may be drawn DOS PM) INR(PT)/APTT	CBC and lytes INR(PT)/APTT	INR(PT)/APTT	INR(PT)/APTT
Other Tests	Hip x-ray Chest x-ray ECG	Portable hip x-ray (PACU or OR)	N/A	Hip x-ray via stretcher if suspect dislocation or subluxation	N/A	N/A
Meds	Prophylactic antibiotic (cephalosporin) at least 1 h before OR PRE-anesthesia meds	Antibiotic IVPB q 6 h x 2–4 doses PCA with meperidine or morphine Antiemetic PRN Coumadin QD or heparin or Lovenox SQ q 8–12 h (contact MD for INR(PT) >3 or APTT >50) Tylenol q 4 h PRN for temp >101°F or pain Stool softener at bedtime	Same as Day 1 (DOS)	Laxative of choice if no BM Same as Day 2 (POD #1) D/C PCA; switch to IM meperidine; Percocet (Tylox) PO q 3–4 h PRN; may use Darvocet-N 100 mg	Continue with PO pain med Stool softener at bedtime Continue with Coumadin/heparin/ Lovenox per MD order based on lab Tylenol PRN for breakthrough pain or fever	Same as Day 4 (POD #3)

Treatments/ Interventions	Betadine scrub (patient may do own)	I & O until IV D/C'd Pillow or abduction splint between legs at all times while in bed Turn patient toward unaffected side with legs abducted TCDB q 2 h; incentive spirometer q 2 h W/A Thigh-high anti-embolism stockings SCDs while in bed ROM to non-operative side Straight cath if not voided 8 h after surgery	I & O Keep legs abducted and turn toward unaffected side TCDB and incentive spirometer q 2 h Thigh-high stockings and SCDs while in bed	Dressing change and drain removal by MD; if healing, may remove dressing Maintain abduction Continue with pulmonary interventions Maintain stockings	Continue with anti-embolism stockings and SCDs Assess skin, especially heels, QD Change dressing BID or clean incision with NS Hip precautions	Same as Day 4 (POD #3)
Nutrition	NPO after 12 midnight	NPO until fully awake, then clear liquids	Full liquids → progress DAT	DAT	Same as Day 3 (POD #2)	Same as Day 4 (POD #3)
Lines/Tubes/ Monitors	N/A	Continuous IV fluids Hemovac or JP drain(s)	Same as Day 1 (DOS)	D/C IV unless vomiting or low Hgb/Hct	N/A	N/A

Figure 7–1. (Continued)

Clinical Pathway for Total Hip Replacement Continued

Aspect of Care (Cont'd)	Date _____ Pre-admission/ Pre-op	Date _____ Day 1 (DOS)	Date _____ Day 2 (POD #1)	Date _____ Day 3 (POD #2)	Date _____ Day 4 (POD #3)	Date _____ Day 5 (POD #4)
Mobility/Self-Care	Activity ad lib	Bed rest/HOB 45° Total care Fracture pan Ankle pumps, quad and gluteal sets Overhead frame/ trapeze on bed	Dangle at bedside, then up in chair with assistance BID using pivot technique Fracture pan/BSC Ankle pumps, quad and gluteal sets Do not hyperflex hips; elevate operative leg when OOB PT for bedside exercises, such as platform walker, if not done pre-op PT evaluation for special needs, if indicated	Up in chair with assistance 2–3 x QD BSC/elevated toilet seat Continue with exercises and hip precautions Same as Day 2 (POD #1)	Up with walker in room BID and PRN with supervision (PWB for cemented prosthesis; toe-touch for noncemented prosthesis) PT BID for progressive ambulation ROM and LE strengthening	Up with walker and into hall 3–4 x QD Continue with PT
Discharge Planning	N/A	Assess home needs and support; financial status	Re-assess home needs and support; collaborate with social worker about possible temporary or permanent placement and financial needs	Same as Day 2 (POD #1)	Continue to collaborate regarding placement into rehab or LTC facility, as needed Involve family/ significant others in discharge planning If discharged to home, refer for home health, PT services	Same as day 4 (POD #3)

Figure 7–1. (Continued)

the nursing home or by the home care agency. By following an individual across the health care continuum, caregivers in each setting know what care has been given, what outcomes have been achieved, and what outcomes still need to be met.

Clinical pathways are fairly new to the long term care setting but have been used in some acute care and home care agencies for more than 10 years. CPs tend to work best for short-term residents and those admitted to subacute care units. Clinical pathways, then, are not appropriate for all residents in long term care. They are typically used for high risk, high volume, high cost resident populations, where they help decrease health care costs by determining what care should be given and when.

If expected outcomes are not met or interventions are not carried out as planned, the nurse documents these deviations from the plan as "variances." Although the pathway is a part of the medical record, the variance documentation is *not* a part of the record. Instead, the variance data are reviewed and analyzed by the facility's quality improvement committee. Trends in variances are identified, and action plans to correct any problems are carried out and followed up by the committee. In other words, the clinical pathway is a quality improvement tool (see Chapter 14 on the quality improvement process).

Progress Notes

Progress notes have traditionally been used by physicians for documenting the resident's health status. Other health care professionals, such as nurses, social workers, and dietitians, used separate chart forms for their documentation.

In recent years, however, many facilities have moved away from this source-oriented approach to the medical record and replaced it with an integrated, problem-oriented approach to documentation to promote communication among members of the health care team. In an integrated medical record, most or all health disciplines chart on the same progress notes. The notes may be organized by an established set of identified resident problems. In some nursing homes, however, nurses still use a separate section of the chart for "nurses' notes."

PURPOSES OF DOCUMENTATION

Documenting resident progress is necessary for several reasons:
1. Legal requirements
2. Reimbursement from third-party payers, such as Medicare
3. Communication among members of the health care team
4. Evidence that quality care was provided

Legal Requirements

According to state nurse practice acts, nurses are required to document the progress of clients in any health care setting using the nursing process. All phases of the nursing process—assessment, analysis (nursing diagnosis), planning, implementation, and evaluation—should be included. In the author's experience as an expert witness for malpractice cases, lack of documented resident assessment is one of the major documentation issues. If the resident's status is not adequately assessed, the nurse may make the wrong decisions about the interventions that are needed for the resident.

For example, if a resident complains of coughing episodes, the nurse may call the health care provider for an order for cough syrup rather than first performing a complete respiratory assessment and vital signs. The medication for cough could mask pneumonia or other respiratory health problems.

In the typical nursing home setting, the frequency of charting on the medical record varies from resident to resident. If the resident's condition has not changed, weekly documentation may be sufficient. If the resident has fallen, charting his or her condition every shift or daily may be appropriate. In a subacute unit, charting every shift is usually required. Table 7–1 lists some important charting tips that help meet the legal requirements for documentation.

Reimbursement from Third-Party Payers

For some residents, the frequency of charting may be somewhat determined by the type of financial reimbursement (payment) for care. For

Table 7–1. **Essential Guidelines for Charting: Dos and Don'ts**

Do:
- Include all phases of the nursing process.
- Write legibly and use correct grammar and spelling.
- Use only dark blue or black nonerasable ink.
- Use specific, descriptive words in a concise manner.
- Date, time, and sign each entry.
- Use resident quotes in charting entries.
- Correct a mistake by writing the word "error" or "mistaken entry" and initial, date, and time correction.
- Use a carat to insert one or two words that were omitted.
- Make a late entry by writing "Late entry for (date, time)" and then write the note.

Don't:
- Leave white space that someone else can write in.
- Erase or use "white-out"; correct mistakes as listed above.
- Block chart (e.g., 7A–3P); rather use the time that the note is entered into the record.
- Use vague terminology or labels, such as "good," "well," "cooperative," and "manipulative."
- Blame others or be judgmental in a note.
- Use "appears" or "apparently"

instance, Medicare pays for skilled care, that is, care performed by a *licensed* health professional. To receive payment for skilled services, the facility must provide documentation that a licensed person was necessary to provide care, rather than a nursing assistant or other unlicensed assistive personnel. Examples of skilled services include daily (5 days a week) physical therapy and nursing care associated with new tube feedings, tracheostomy, and intravenous therapy. Most insurance companies that provide Medicare funds, called intermediaries, prefer at least daily charting regarding the skilled service.

State-administered medical assistance programs (such as Medicaid) for those who cannot afford care also require documentation that certain aspects of care have been provided. For example, in most states, the residents' ability to perform activities of daily living must be documented at periodic intervals. For bed bound residents, turning and repositioning must be documented every 2 hours. The rules governing the charting requirements for residents receiving medical assistance, which vary state by state, must be adhered to for payment.

Communication among Health Team Members

Resident care in a nursing home requires an interdisciplinary approach. Therefore, it is extremely important that members of the health care team communicate verbally as well as in the medical record. Each member should read what other team members have written in the chart. Documenting on the same progress notes helps to facilitate this process, because all information about the resident is in one place.

Evidence of Quality Care

The old adage that "if it wasn't documented, it wasn't done" is perhaps a safe rule to live by. While the courts now recognize that health professionals sometimes forget to chart important observations and interventions, the best way to prove that quality care was provided is to document that care.

In this author's experience, most nurses seem to dislike charting because they find it time-consuming and redundant at times. They often chart at the end of their shift, which results in inadequate or faulty documentation. Instead of viewing documentation as an additional task after the care is completed, it is probably best to think of charting as the most important aspect of resident care. If a nurse provides excellent care but does not document it, no one else will know what care was rendered.

Another reason to document care is for chart review that may be done at a later time for quality improvement (QI) studies, chart audits, or research. In each of these cases, the person who reviews the chart looks for evidence of quality care provided by the interdisciplinary health team.

For example, the QI coordinator may be concerned with the incidence of pressure ulcers on a nursing unit. The first step in this study would be to review charts to determine how many pressure ulcers occurred in the unit and who was most at risk for developing the ulcers. The coordinator would also want to look at how many residents were admitted with existing pressure ulcers acquired before admission to the facility.

METHODS OF CHARTING RESIDENT PROGRESS

The methods that nurses use to document care in the medical record have changed over the past 20 years. While a number of charting systems are still used in nursing homes, three systems seem to be the most popular:

1. Narrative charting
2. PIE charting
3. Focus charting

Narrative Charting

Narrative charting is the most traditional form of documentation. Using this method, the nurse records the care in chronological order, describing what happened first, second, and so forth. The note typically consists of assorted sentences, phrases, and clauses, strung together by commas, colons, dashes, and periods.

The advantage of narrative notes is that they provide a story or summary along a time line. Nurses who have used this form of charting usually feel comfortable with it.

The disadvantages of narrative charting, however, may outweigh the advantages. For instance, narrative notes often include information that is useless or meaningless, such as "Resident had a good day," "Visitors in this afternoon," or "Watching TV." None of these statements tells anything about the resident's condition or fits into any of the phases of the nursing process.

Another disadvantage is the inability to easily find information. Many of the resident's health problems are discussed in a single note. Other health team members may not read this type of chart entry because it is difficult to follow and often includes meaningless information that no one has the time to read.

PIE Charting

PIE charting is one of several charting methods that provide a problem-oriented approach to documentation. In a PIE note, the nurse records information related to **P** for Problem, **I** for Interventions, and **E** for Evaluation. Figure 7–2 shows a sample PIE note for a typical resident

```
2/7/97----------------P: Athritic pain in both knees; no swelling or
11:15 AM --------------------redness.-----------------------------------------
------------------------I : Gave Tylenol tabs ii @ 10:20 AM. Reminded to
--------------------------------use walker when ambulating.-----------------
------------------------E: States that medication has "eased the worst of
--------------------------------the pain."-----------------------------------------
------------------------------------------------------------------Sue Smith, RNC
```

Figure 7–2. *PIE charting.*

health problem in a nursing home. The problem that labels the note may come from a master problem list found in the medical record.

A variation of the PIE note is the APIE note, which adds Assessment to the steps of the nursing process for complete documentation. For **A**, the nurse documents the subjective data (what the resident or family says) and the objective data (what the nurse measures, observes, or palpates related to the problem label).

The major advantage of the PIE or APIE system is that all phases of the nursing process are recorded and are associated with individual resident health problems. All of the information is meaningful and easy to find and follow. The disadvantage of this type of system is that it is a major change in the way that nurses have traditionally charted. A comprehensive educational process is needed to help nurses concentrate on the steps of the nursing process as they chart.

Focus Charting

Focus charting was initiated in the acute care setting in an attempt to streamline and organize documentation but can easily be used in long term care. In some ways, focus charting is similar to the PIE approach in that it identifies residents' problems or concerns and forces the writer to concentrate on the steps of the nursing process. As shown in Figure 7–3, the progress or nurses' note is divided in half. The left side of the paper is the column for the problem, concern, or need, and is entitled "Focus." On the right side, the information related to the focus is charted using a DAR system. **D** stands for data (both subjective and objective); **A** stands for action; and **R** stands for response. Like the **E** in the PIE method, the evaluation of the action or intervention may not be known until a later time, as seen in Figure 7–3.

The advantage of the focus charting method is its structure, which forces the writer to be specific and write only the information needed. The information in the resident's chart can be easily located using this system. Focus charting also avoids the use of a set master problem list because a focus can be a need or concern. For example, an abnormal lab value may not be an actual problem but needs to be documented because it could become a problem and requires monitoring.

```
                 FOCUS                              NOTE
3/2/97---------------Fever--------------------------------D: Temp. 100.6 (o) @ 12N.
1 PM----------------------------------------------------------Face flushed and warm.
------------------------------------------------------------c/o dry mouth-------------
------------------------------------------------------------A: Continue plan of care
------------------------------------------------------------including Tylenol
------------------------------------------------------------tabs ii q4h if temp.
------------------------------------------------------------above 100.8. Pushing
------------------------------------------------------------fluids; has had 600 mL
------------------------------------------------------------over last 2 h.---------------
------------------------------------------------------------R: Temp. decreased since 8AM;
------------------------------------------------------------plan effective in reducing
------------------------------------------------------------fever. Donna Jenkins, LPN
```

Figure 7–3. Focus charting.

The disadvantage of the focus charting method is the need for education and support to help nurses use a system that is very different from the traditional narrative method. The focus method also takes more space on paper because the actual note is confined to the right half of the page.

Skin Assessment Record

In most nursing homes, a separate "skin sheet" is used to document skin problems (skin lesions), such as pressure ulcers, unexplained bruises, rashes, and skin tears. Most skin assessment records have a line drawing of a person with both the anterior and posterior views to allow the nurse to draw the precise location of the skin lesion. The remainder of the document has a section where the nurse can chart the date, time, and description of the skin lesion. If more than one skin problem is present, each is assigned a number or letter. In most nursing home settings, the skin sheet is updated at least once per week. Weekly charting may not be sufficient, however, for deep wounds, which may need observation and documentation three times a week or daily.

Medication Administration Record

The medication administration record (MAR) used in nursing homes is not unlike those used in other health care settings. Typically, each resident has two MARs—one for routine or regimen drugs and the other for "as needed," or PRN, drugs. The PRN medication record in a nursing home usually has a place to record the date, time, drug, dose, and reason for medication administration. Another column to record the results of the medication may also be part of the MAR. For example, if an analgesic is given for arthritic pain, the nurse needs to evaluate the resident about an hour after the medication is given to evaluate whether or not the medication was effective in relieving the pain. In other words, the nurse evaluates the resident to determine if the expected outcome was met and documents the findings.

Each drug listed on both MARs should have a reason why the drug has been ordered, for example, "Digoxin 0.125 mg QD for atrial fibrillation." The stated purpose for the medication is to ensure that the resident receives only the necessary drugs, as per the federal Omnibus Budget Reconciliation Act (OBRA) (see Chapters 5 and 13 for a discussion of this topic).

Activity and Treatment Record

Many activities and treatments for nursing home residents are performed every day on a routine basis. Rather than repeatedly document the treatment in the progress notes, a flow sheet, similar to the format of the MAR, is used. The nurse documents that the activity or treatment was completed by writing his or her initials in the appropriate space.

Incident Report

The incident report is a document that is *not* kept on the resident's chart. Rather it is an internal document that is reviewed by the risk management (or designee) or quality improvement coordinator and/or committee for the purpose of identifying actual or potential problems in resident care. The incident report is used to record any unusual occurrence, such as a resident fall or medication error. Some facilities use a separate form for medication errors. The follow-up investigation or analysis is also kept as an internal record and therefore should be kept in a locked file.

When completing the incident report, the nurse should follow the legal guidelines that include important "dos" and "don'ts" (Table 7–2), just as in charting on the medical record.

Table 7–2. Essential Guidelines for Completing Incident Reports

- Don't write in the medical record that an incident report has been completed or filed.
- Be sure that the information in the chart and the incident report is the same.
- Don't blame others or be judgmental in the incident report.
- Don't discuss how the incident could have been avoided or what the follow-up investigation was on the incident report form.
- Use concise, specific words to describe the incident.
- Use dark blue or black ink.
- Keep incident reports in a secure, locked area and do not photocopy for distribution.

CHAPTER HIGHLIGHTS

A comprehensive, interdisciplinary resident care plan is required for every resident in a nursing home.

Clinical pathways are predetermined guidelines for care that outline optimum sequencing of interventions across a time line.

Documentation of the resident's progress is needed for:

1. Legal requirements
2. Reimbursement by third-party payers
3. Communication among the health care team
4. Evidence that quality care was provided

Three methods of charting resident progress are narrative notes, PIE charting, and focus charting.

The skin assessment record is used to document the presence and progress of rashes, bruises, and wounds.

The activity and treatment record is used to document routine or repeated activities and treatments performed for residents.

An incident report is an internal document used to study trends for actual or potential problems in the delivery of resident care; the incident report is *not* kept on the resident's medical record.

REFERENCES AND READINGS

Better documentation. (1992). Springhouse, PA: Springhouse.

Fischbach, F. T. (1991). *Documenting care: Communication, the nursing process and documentation standards.* Philadelphia: F. A. Davis.

Ignatavicius, D. D. (1988). Documentation: The essence of client care. *Focus on Geriatric Care and Rehabilitation.*

Ignatavicius, D. D., & Hausman, K. (1995). *Clinical pathways for collaborative practice.* Philadelphia: W. B. Saunders.

Iyer, P. W., & Camp, N. H. (1991). *Nursing documentation: A nursing process approach.* St. Louis: Mosby Year Book.

Lampe, S. (1988). *Focus charting.* Minneapolis: Creative Nursing Management.

DISCUSSION QUESTIONS TO PROMOTE CRITICAL THINKING

1. What are the advantages of the PIE and focus charting systems as compared to the traditional narrative charting?

2. You receive a laboratory report that shows one of your residents has a low potassium level. He has been on diuretics for many years. Write a note that illustrates this information and your action using the focus charting format.

3. A resident has repeated skin tears because her skin is extremely thin from chronic steroid therapy for her rheumatoid arthritis. The staff complains that they often complete four to six incident reports a day regarding skin tears. Because the purpose of the incident report is to track actual or potential care problems, is it necessary for the nurses to complete an incident report on every tear? Why or why not?

8

Health Protection and Promotion in the Nursing Home

OBJECTIVES

- Describe the relationship of health promotion and health protection
- State two reasons why health promotion and protection are needed for residents in the nursing home
- Identify at least three factors that should be assessed as part of the teaching-learning process
- List at least six tips for teaching elderly residents in the nursing home

Health *promotion* is a broad term that refers to various activities directed at enhancing wellness. *Health protection* (illness prevention) can be considered a type of health promotion in that it involves activities that prevent illness. Both health promotion and protection activities reduce health care costs because they aim to keep people healthy in the community, thus reducing the need for health care services. In addition, an individual's quality of life and functional ability are improved through health promotion efforts.

The increased incidence of chronic diseases, such as cancer and heart disease, in people over 65 years of age supports the need for a shift to health protection and health promotion for the elderly. The emphasis in nursing homes has traditionally been on illness rather than wellness, although this focus is changing.

The nature of residents in the nursing home is also changing. First, as described earlier in this book, younger residents—those under 65— are being admitted to nursing homes for chronic diseases and disabilities, such as multiple sclerosis and spinal cord injury. Second, the length of stay for many nursing home residents is very short, often 1 to 4 weeks. Third, the long-term resident in the nursing home is living longer with a higher quality of life than in previous years. Each of these changes influences the need for strategies for health promotion, as well as concern for illness care.

Healthy People 2000

The U.S. Department of Health and Human Services (1990) outlined objectives (goals) for improving health among adults age 65 and older in its *Healthy People 2000* document. Examples of these objectives are listed in Table 8–1. Nursing home staff have an opportunity to help meet these goals through resident education and early detection of health problems.

Resident Education

Nurses have been taught the importance of health teaching through formal and continuing education programs, but they often feel that they do not

Table 8–1. **Sample Health Promotion Objectives for People 65 and Older**

Increase:
- Immunization levels for pneumonia and influenza among the elderly, especially the chronically ill elderly
- The percentage of older adults who regularly participate in light to moderate activity for at least 30 minutes a day
- Years of healthy life to at least 65 among blacks and Hispanics

Reduce:
- Significant visual impairment
- Suicide among white men
- Death from falls and fall-related injury
- Hip fractures
- Epidemic-related pneumonia and influenza deaths

From U.S. Department of Health and Human Services (1990).

have the time to implement this intervention. In addition, some residents in nursing homes are severely demented or have other impairments that make teaching difficult. However, many short-term and younger residents, as well as families of all residents, can benefit from teaching.

TEACHING-LEARNING PRINCIPLES

The teaching-learning process follows the steps of the nursing process. First, the nurse, in collaboration with the health team, *assesses* the resident's and family's knowledge level; the factors affecting learning, such as culture, motivation, and educational level; the resident's readiness to learn; and available support systems.

The health team should not assume that a resident who has had a chronic disease for a long time understands the condition and the care required. The resident may not be motivated or ready to learn. Individuals diagnosed with chronic illness must work through the grieving process before they are ready to learn about the illness. Then, the nurse can *analyze* what they already know and still need to know.

The *planning* and *implementation* phases of the teaching-learning process can be the most difficult steps because the nurse needs to select an appropriate environment and appropriate teaching method that will be conducive to learning. Usually, the best time to teach an elderly resident is early in the morning, after breakfast. At that time the resident is not fatigued, and residents are often more lucid in the morning than in the late afternoon or evening. If the resident wears glasses, contact lenses, or a hearing aid, these devices must be in place to facilitate the resident's understanding.

The elderly may take a little longer to learn, but they are able to learn new information at any age. In some cases, the information may need to be repeated or reinforced with visual aids, such as pictures. Teaching the resident in a quiet place prevents distractions that could interfere with learning.

Resident education can be divided into formal and informal teaching. Formal teaching typically involves a structured program presented in modules or sections, such as that used for cardiac rehabilitation, diabetic teaching, or discharge planning. Informal teaching is often unplanned, such as when the resident asks about the purpose of a medication and the nurse answers the question at that time.

The teaching-learning process should use an interdisciplinary approach when feasible. For example, the physical therapist may initially teach the resident how to use a cane, but the nurse needs to reinforce the learning and evaluate whether or not the resident understood the instructions. This example illustrates the last step of the teaching-learning process, which is *evaluation.*

The nurse or other health professional can provide excellent teaching, but the most important step of the teaching-learning process is to ensure

Table 8–2. **Tips for Teaching Elderly Nursing Home Residents**

- Assess the environment to determine if it is conducive to learning; it should be quiet, private, and free of distractions.
- Assess the resident's readiness and motivation to learn.
- Assess the resident for cultural factors and educational background that may impact learning ability.
- Include the family and/or significant others in health teaching.
- Ensure that the resident and family are comfortable before teaching.
- Ensure that the resident wears glasses and hearing aids, if appropriate.
- Use an interdisciplinary approach to the teaching-learning process.
- Teach residents in the morning, when possible.
- Use visual aids and demonstration, as appropriate, to reinforce verbal teaching.
- Set realistic goals for teaching; teach content in small amounts.
- Encourage questions from both the resident and family.
- Evaluate whether learning has occurred.
- Document all resident education interventions and response to the teaching-learning process.

that the resident and family have learned the information and changed behavior as a result of the educational process. Asking the resident to restate what was learned or to demonstrate care are examples of evaluation. Observing resident behavior, such as selecting foods from a menu or self-administering insulin, reveals whether or not the resident has learned these aspects of care. Table 8–2 lists tips for health teaching in the nursing home.

INTERVENTIONS FOR HEALTH PROTECTION

Health protection, also called illness prevention, means that the interdisciplinary team uses strategies, especially health teaching, to help residents prevent further episodes of an illness or complications of an illness. For example, a resident who has experienced a myocardial infarction (MI) can reduce the risk of another MI by following certain guidelines, including stress reduction, diet restrictions, and regular exercise. The diabetic resident needs to learn about the importance of skin and foot care, avoiding infections, and complying with an American Diabetes Association (ADA) diet.

Specific teaching-learning needs and interventions should be listed on the interdisciplinary resident care plan or clinical pathway (see Chapter 7). In some agencies, a teaching-learning resident education guide is also used. The nurse or other health team member initials each area taught to the resident, then evaluates whether or not the resident has assimilated the information in the column provided.

INTERVENTIONS FOR HEALTH PROMOTION

In addition to health protection, the focus for resident education is the need for other health promotion strategies. Appendix E describes common complementary therapies that can be used by residents or nurses to promote health and healing using the body-mind-spirit connection.

All residents should receive diagnostic testing, monitoring, or immunizations for illnesses that typically occur in the elderly or chronically ill. These interventions to promote health have typically not been implemented in nursing homes across the United States. In keeping with the goals of *Healthy People 2000*, however, health promotion needs to be a major focus of nursing homes. Nurses, in particular, have been taught to promote health as a major focus for health care.

Respiratory Infections

Influenza and pneumonia are major infections that kill many elderly and chronically ill individuals every year. Immunizations for influenza and pneumonia are readily available and should be administered to residents living in the nursing home, as well as those residing in the community.

Residents who have acquired these infections should be kept away from healthy residents. The same principle applies for any infection that can be spread from resident to resident.

Cancer

Cancer is another disease that primarily affects the elderly. Over half of all cancers occur in people over 65 (American Cancer Society [ACS], 1995). Screening and early detection increase the chance for a cure in most cases; yet screening and detection programs are not common in the nursing home industry. Table 8–3 lists the recommendations by the ACS regarding screening and early detection of cancer in individuals 65 and older.

If the resident is unable to be taught how to perform breast self-examination, testicular self-examination, or skin self-examination as recommended, the nursing staff should be instructed on these techniques. The staff should check areas of the skin that the resident cannot see, such

Table 8–3. **American Cancer Society Guidelines for Early Detection of Cancer in People 65 and Older**

Examination	Schedule
Complete physical examination	Every year
Pelvic examination (with Pap smear)	Every year
Mammogram	Every year
Digital rectal examination	Every year
Stool for occult blood	Every year
Prostate-specific antigen testing	Every year
Breast self-examination	Every month
Sigmoidoscopy	Every 3–5 yrs

as the back and buttocks. If caught early, skin cancer is almost always curable. Melanoma is the most serious skin cancer and can be differentiated from a mole by using the ABCD rule: A melanoma is *asymmetrical* (uneven), the *border* is irregular, the *color* is mixed, and the *diameter* is larger than a pencil eraser.

Osteoporosis

Some residents are more likely to acquire health problems than others. For instance, petite, postmenopausal Caucasian women are at a very high risk of osteoporosis. Osteoporosis is a disease in which bones become porous and fracture due to decreased estrogen levels. Unfortunately, a diagnosis of osteoporosis is not typically made until the woman falls and breaks a bone, often a hip. For this population at risk, the health team can teach about the importance of consuming foods high in calcium, such as dairy products and green, leafy vegetables; the need to decrease caffeine and smoking; and the need for calcium supplements, perhaps in combination with hormone replacement therapy (HRT) and vitamin D. While these measures may not totally prevent osteoporosis, they tend to slow the progression of the disease.

CHAPTER HIGHLIGHTS

The emphasis in nursing homes has traditionally been on illness rather than wellness, although this focus is changing.

The teaching-learning process follows the steps of the nursing process.

Health teaching should involve the interdisciplinary team.

Health protection, also called illness prevention, helps residents prevent further episodes of an illness or complications of an illness, such as diabetes mellitus.

Health promotion involves diagnostic testing, monitoring, and immunizations for illnesses that typically occur in the elderly or chronically ill, such as the pneumonia vaccine.

REFERENCES AND READINGS

Alford, D. M., & Futrell, M. (1992). Wellness and health promotion of the elderly. *Nursing Outlook, 40*, 221–226.

American Cancer Society. (1995). *Cancer facts and figures—1995*. Atlanta: Author.

Bigbee, J. L., & Jansa, N. (1991). Strategies for promoting health protection. *Nursing Clinics of North America, 26*, 895–913.

Spellbring, A. M. (1991). Nursing's role in health promotion. *Nursing Clinics of North America, 26*, 805–814.

U.S. Department of Health and Human Services, Public Health Service. (1990). *Healthy people 2000: National health promotion and disease prevention objectives*. Washington, DC: U.S. Government Printing Office.

DISCUSSION QUESTIONS TO PROMOTE CRITICAL THINKING

1. Why should there be more emphasis on health promotion and health protection in the nursing home setting?

2. In what ways could geriatric nursing assistants help with health promotion and protection activities?

3. What special health teaching needs might younger residents have?

Subacute Care

OBJECTIVES

- Define subacute care
- Identify two accreditations that subacute care units often seek
- Describe three types of subacute care units
- Discuss the skills that subacute care nurses need
- Briefly define the role of the case manager in subacute care

Subacute (SA) care, sometimes called transitional care, is the newest level of health care for individuals who no longer need hospital care but are too ill to be discharged to a traditional nursing home or their own home. Therefore, SA care is sometimes referred to as "filling the gap" between acute care and long term care.

During the past several years, SA care has grown tremendously. In 1995 the market size was estimated at $1.4 billion. The prediction for 1997 is

$2.7 billion. About one-third of health care services offered in subacute units are rehabilitation services; the remainder are medical-surgical services (Stahl, 1994).

The growth of subacute care is related to the expansion of managed care—insurance-based strategies designed to provide cost-effective quality health care, such as that provided by health maintenance organizations (HMOs). Subacute units have developed in less than half of the United States. Most are located in freestanding nursing homes. A smaller number are located in hospitals.

Definitions of Subacute Care

The American Health Care Association (AHCA), the leading representative of the long term care industry, defines subacute care as a "comprehensive inpatient program designed for the individual who has had an acute event as a result of an illness, injury, or exacerbation [flare-up] of a disease process; has a determined course of treatment; and does not require intensive diagnostic and/or invasive procedures" (American Health Care Association, 1994).

Another popular definition was published by the Joint Commission on Accreditation of Healthcare Organizations (JCAHO), the voluntary accreditation agency for hospitals and other health care settings. This organization gathered a panel of subacute care experts, Healthcare professionals, and consumers to develop their definition. Like the AHCA, JCAHO also defines subacute care as comprehensive inpatient care designed for an individual who has had an acute illness, injury, or disease exacerbation. Both organizations further stress the need for coordinated care using an interdisciplinary approach.

Standards and Regulations Governing Subacute Care

Managed care organizations (MCOs) are eagerly seeking to contract with subacute units to provide services for their clients to save the high cost of hospital care. These MCOs usually require that their subacute units be accredited by JCAHO.

ACCREDITATION BY THE JOINT COMMISSION ON ACCREDITATION OF HEALTHCARE ORGANIZATIONS

As a result of the request for JCAHO accreditation and the need to have standards which assure that subacute units are providing high quality care, JCAHO published its standards for SA care in January 1995. A subacute unit that applies for accreditation by JCAHO must first be surveyed using the long term care (LTC) standards. If the SA unit passes the LTC survey, it then must pass the SA survey. The SA survey usually takes about 2 days. The cost of the survey depends on the number of unit beds.

In addition to the JCAHO survey, the unit is also surveyed by each state's licensing and certification agency to ensure that the unit is meeting the federal and state regulations that were described in Chapter 2. The state survey is mandated by law, whereas the JCAHO survey is a voluntary accreditation.

COMMISSION ON ACCREDITATION OF REHABILITATION FACILITIES

If the SA unit has a rehabilitation focus, it may also want accreditation by the Commission for Accreditation of Rehabilitation Facilities (CARF). This organization surveys all types of rehabilitation units and hospitals. The CARF survey for SA units usually takes about 2 days at a cost of almost $3000. Like the JCAHO accreditation, this is a voluntary accreditation demonstrating to the public that the subacute unit is fully qualified to provide quality health care to its residents.

Settings for Subacute Care

The majority of SA units are currently located in freestanding nursing homes that are affiliated with large corporations. The nursing home must have one or more distinct units designated for skilled care. Skilled care requires that care be provided by health care professionals, such as nurses, physical therapists, and occupational therapists. The corporation or individual facility decides what type of residents it will admit to the subacute unit based on community need, financial resources, human resources, and other factors. A study of the market's needs (feasibility study) helps determine this need.

Many hospitals have experienced a decreasing patient census as a result of having discharged patients more quickly to reduce costs. Some hospitals have converted one or more patient care units to subacute care in an effort to utilize the beds, make money, and provide a place where their patients can go after the acute care phase. Another advantage of hospital-based subacute care is the smooth transition from one level of care to another—a "seamless" transfer between levels of care, as required by JCAHO. The staff can readily communicate with one another and ensure continuity of care within the same institution.

Types of Subacute Care Patients

When individuals are admitted to hospital-based SA care, they may be referred to as patients or residents. Many prefer to be called patients, implying a short length of stay. When they are admitted to SA units in nursing homes, they are usually called residents. The term *resident* implies that the individual is residing in a homelike environment, rather than in an institution.

Regardless of location for SA care, each unit must decide what type of residents it will admit. Will the unit be specialized and accept only one type of resident? Examples include ventilator-dependent residents for a "vent" unit and brain-injured residents for a traumatic brain injury (TBI) unit. These individuals require very high level care and special physical plant considerations. For example, if the unit does not have the environmental requirements (such as emergency electrical power) to use certain equipment, such as ventilators, then the unit is limited in the type of resident it can accept.

More commonly, most subacute units accept several types of residents. These residents can be grouped into three major categories: transitional subacute, general medical-surgical subacute, and long-term transitional subacute (Table 9–1).

Table 9–1. **Categories of Subacute Care**

Definition of Category	Examples of Admissions
Transitional Subacute Care A substitute or alternative for continued hospital stays	Deep wound management Stroke rehabilitation Vascular or cardiac surgery Oncology surgery with chemotherapy Medically complex care Complicated orthopedic surgery
Medical-Surgical Subacute Care A setting for stable residents who require moderate level of care	Uncomplicated orthopedic surgery Individuals with HIV Intravenous therapy Uncomplicated tracheostomy care Stroke rehabilitation
Long-Term Transitional Subacute Care A setting for medically complex residents	Acute ventilator support Medically complex residents requiring an extended stay

* Data from Stahl, D. A. (1994).

TRANSITIONAL SUBACUTE CARE

Transitional subacute care (sometimes referred to as a transitional care unit, or TCU) serves as a substitute for continued hospital care. Examples include deep wound management, cardiac care following myocardial infarction or heart surgery, rehabilitation for strokes or complicated orthopedic surgery, and complex care for diabetes, gastrointestinal disorders, and renal disease. Residents in transitional subacute units receive intense, high level care and may be discharged to home or an alternate setting, such as a traditional nursing home unit, in 7 to 12 days.

MEDICAL-SURGICAL SUBACUTE CARE

Like transitional care, medical-surgical subacute care accepts residents with a variety of health problems. These residents, however, are usually more stable and require a shorter stay in the SA unit. Examples include rehabilitation for uncomplicated orthopedic surgery, continued rehabilitation for strokes, individuals with HIV, and others requiring episodic intravenous therapy. Residents are usually discharged to home or assisted-living facilities.

LONG-TERM TRANSITIONAL SUBACUTE CARE

Long-term transitional subacute care units provide care for medically complex residents or those requiring acute ventilator support. Medical and nursing specialists are needed to implement the treatment plan. Residents receive a high level of care in these units.

The Role of the Nurse in Subacute Care

Little has been written about the role of the nurse in subacute care or the staffing requirements for nurses in these settings. Obviously, the number and type of staff depend on the type of resident admitted to the unit and the severity and acuity of the health problems. In general, the staffing on a SA unit is at least 1½ to 2 times that of a traditional unit.

Nurses who work in subacute care must be knowledgable about long term care. They must also have medical-surgical, critical care, and/or rehabilitation skills. For a ventilator-dependent unit, a critical care nurse with Advanced Certification in Life Support (ACLS) may be required. (Respiratory therapy must also be available 24 hours a day.) A rehabilitation unit may require nurses certified in that field.

Regardless of the type of SA care, few nurses have a background that has provided them with all of the skills needed to work in subacute care.

Nursing homes and hospitals employing SA care nurses are responsible for educating them to ensure that they have the necessary skills to provide quality care.

Internal Case Management in Subacute Care

Case management has been available in community settings and as an insurance-based concept for a number of years. Case managers—usually nurses—hired by insurance companies evaluate patients with rehabilitation and subacute health problems to determine what they will pay the agency for care. This type of case management is referred to as external case management.

Internal case management is a fairly new concept to health care. In this sense, case management is a practice model using a systematic approach to identify specific patients and manage patient care to ensure patient outcomes. Case management plays a major role in managed care because it ensures that the best possible care will be provided in a cost-effective manner.

The case manager, most often a nurse employed by the agency, coordinates care provided by the interdisciplinary team, a key concept in the delivery of subacute care. Because the case manager is a care coordinator, case management has also been called coordinated care, collaborative care, and care management.

In addition to the importance of the interdisciplinary team approach is the need to coordinate care across health care settings. For example, the case manager (CM) in subacute care works closely with the CM in acute care as well as the CM in the setting to which the patient is discharged. In some situations, the same CM, usually hospital-based, follows the patient across all of these settings.

THE NURSE AS CASE MANAGER

Nurses were the first to develop case management models for use in hospitals and other settings as a way to deliver consistent coordinated care that decreased the individual's length of stay in the health care setting. Karen Zander and her colleagues are credited with the first nursing case management system at the New England Medical Center. Since the development of her model more than 10 years ago, case management has evolved and encompasses a variety of specific models.

In the subacute unit, the unit-based model may be the most effective because the unit is confined and distinct from other parts of the health care facility, usually a nursing home or hospital. As shown in Figure 9–1, a sub-

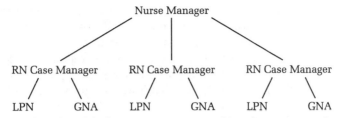

Figure 9–1. *Unit-based model of case management used in subacute care units.*

acute unit may have several case managers who coordinate care for a group of residents. One method of dividing the case load may be to match the type of subacute care being provided with the expertise of the case manager. For example, a certified rehabilitation nurse may be the case manager for the residents receiving rehabilitative services, and the certified medical-surgical or critical care nurse may be the case manager for the other residents.

In most subacute care units, the primary role of the the case manager is to coordinate care, as well as to assist in direct care responsibilities. Although the qualifications for the case manager vary depending on the type of subacute care, many units require a baccalaureate-prepared registered nurse with the appropriate certifications. In some agencies, a master's degree in nursing with a clinical specialty may be required.

CLINICAL PATHWAYS AS A TOOL FOR CASE MANAGEMENT

As discussed in Chapter 7, the interdisciplinary care plan is an important document in the nursing home for long term care residents. In case managed subacute settings, especially those in which the length of stay is short, the clinical pathway serves as the interdisciplinary plan of care. Clinical pathways are guidelines that outline the sequencing of interventions to assist the resident in achieving predetermined optimal outcomes. The case manager ensures that the resident is progressing according to the pathway and documents deviations, or variances, that may occur. Chapter 7 discusses clinical pathways in detail.

Future of Subacute Care

Subacute care continues to expand across the country. People are being discharged "quicker and sicker" from the hospital in an attempt to save money. Many patients continue to need some level of inpatient care.

Currently much of the cost of subacute care is reimbursed by Medicare. The individual is transferred from a hospital where a 3-day qualifying stay allows Medicare to pay for continued skilled care. In the future, legislation may allow an individual to be admitted directly to a subacute care unit for care, rather than be transferred from acute care.

Capitation is another concept that has begun to change the way that health care is reimbursed. In a capitated system, the facility receives a set amount of money for care of each patient or resident per month or other time frame. The facility or unit decides how that money is to be used to meet the expected outcomes. Regardless of how subacute care and reimbursement take shape in the future, the focus on outcomes will be the mainstay of care. Nurses will need to concentrate on helping residents meet outcomes, rather than focus on daily nursing tasks and activities, as was done in the past.

CHAPTER HIGHLIGHTS

As a result of the expansion of managed care, subacute care is the fastest growing segment of the health care industry.

Subacute care "fills the gap" between acute care and long term care.

Subacute care is a comprehensive inpatient program for individuals who have had an acute illness, injury, or disease exacerbation.

Subacute units must pass their state long term care survey; they may also apply for voluntary accreditation by the Joint Commission on the Accreditation of Healthcare Organizations and the Commission on the Accreditation of Rehabilitation Facilities.

Subacute units may be located in freestanding nursing homes (most common) or in hospitals.

The types of subacute care may be broadly categorized as transitional subacute, medical-surgical subacute, and long-term transitional subacute care.

Nurses who work in subacute care must have a wide range of skills related to medical-surgical, critical care, and long term care nursing.

Internal case management is an important part of subacute care; it is a practice model that ensures that care is coordinated using an interdisciplinary approach.

Case managers, usually nurses, use clinical pathways as guidelines for planning care in a case management system.

REFERENCES AND READINGS

American Health Care Association. (1994). *Blueprint for the future vision.* Washington, DC: Author.

Brown-Goebeler, S. (1994). Subacute care: Nursing for the next century. *MEDSURG Nursing, 3,* 497–499.

Hyatt, L. (1995). *Subacute care: Redefining health care.* Burr Ridge, IL: Irwin Professional Publishing.

Stahl, D. A. (1994). Subacute care: The future of health care. *Nursing Management, 25* (10), 34–40.

Walsh, G. G. (1995). How subacute care fills the gap. *Nursing 95, 25* (3), 51.

DISCUSSION QUESTIONS TO PROMOTE CRITICAL THINKING

1. What specific types of skills do you think a nurse needs to work on a subacute unit?
2. What is the benefit of case management for the subacute unit?
3. Why is subacute care expected to grow into the twenty-first century?

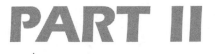

PART II

THE NURSE'S ROLE AS MANAGER IN LONG TERM CARE

10 Philosophy and Structure of the Nursing Home

OBJECTIVES

- Identify three basic types of ownership for nursing homes
- Identify the primary role of the nursing home administrator
- Describe the roles of clinical departments, including physician services and the nursing department
- Describe the role of nonclinical departments, including quality improvement and staff development
- Identify at least one consultant role in the nursing home setting

Although the concept of long term care is similar across the nation, individual differences distinguish one nursing facility from another. This chapter describes the ownership and departmental structure of nursing homes.

Role of Ownership

Each nursing home is set up differently depending on its ownership structure. Most facilities are for-profit homes, meaning that the facility needs to make a profit to stay in business. A smaller number of nursing homes are not-for-profit or nonprofit facilities. Not-for-profit nursing homes are not established for the purpose of making money, but they would prefer to make money rather than lose money. Nonprofit homes may not make a profit and therefore all revenues are invested back into the facility. Still other nursing homes are owned and operated by federal, state, or county governments.

FOR-PROFIT OWNERSHIP

The ownership of private, for-profit facilities is set up in a variety of ways. Independent, private nursing homes are those that have one owner or a small group of owners who invest in the facility. These are often partnership arrangements.

Some nursing homes are part of a chain of homes, that is, a small or large corporation owns a number of facilities. Examples of the largest corporations in the United States that own nursing homes are Beverly, Hillhaven, Manor Care, and Genesis. Some of the large corporations offer stock to the public to bolster their financial position. The governing body of a corporation, the board of directors, has the legal responsibility for the operation of the corporation. If the corporation is public, stockholders receive dividends on their investment in the company.

NOT-FOR-PROFIT AND NONPROFIT OWNERSHIP

Most nonprofit nursing homes are owned and operated by churches. Like a corporation, these facilities typically have a board of directors that oversees the fiscal (financial) and operational aspects of one or more nursing homes. They usually do not have stockholders who invest in the facilities.

GOVERNMENT OWNERSHIP

Long term care facilities may be owned and/or operated by city, county, state, or federal governments. County homes are the most common. Taxpayers support the operation of a county home, and its governing body, such as the county commission, oversees its operation. Many local and state governments are finding that it is too costly to run a nursing home and are selling their facilities to the private sector.

The Veterans Administration operates a number of nursing homes around the country for veterans. Federal funds support the care of veterans in these facilities.

MISSION AND PHILOSOPHY OF NURSING HOMES

Whether or not a nursing home is part of a corporation or it is an independent facility, all nursing homes strive to provide excellent resident care in a cost-effective manner. Most homes have mission statements that describe how each facility intends to meet that goal. Chapter 2 discusses the mission of nursing homes and identifies the various types of facilities that exist today.

Role of the Nursing Home Administrator

The nursing home administrator (NHA) is responsible for overseeing the day-to-day operations of the nursing home and is accountable to the ownership, whether an individual or a group of individuals, or to a board of directors. The primary role of the NHA is to ensure that the care rendered is of high quality and is cost-effective, staying within budgetary limits while meeting current federal, state, and local standards.

Although state requirements for NHAs vary somewhat, many states require that the individual must have a baccalaureate degree, preferably in health care management or business administration, and a license earned from the state in which the NHA is employed. The procedure for obtaining a license also varies but usually requires that the candidate take a recognized NHA course and be precepted as an "administrator-in-training" (AIT) for 6 to 12 months. After completion of this training, the candidate must pass a state and federal examination to earn a license for practice in that state. Each state has a board of nursing home administrators that governs NHA practice. Like nurses, NHAs can be disciplined by their board and are accountable for their practice. For example, if substandard care is cited in a nursing home survey, it can be reported to the board for possible action.

Role of Clinical Departments

A number of departments report to the NHA. Most of the departments provide direct ("hands-on") resident care. These are sometimes referred to as clinical departments. Other departments support the function of the nursing home but are not responsible for direct care. All departments are needed to meet the needs of the residents and to comply with state and federal regulations.

The major focus of nursing home care is the resident as well as the family or signficant others. The members of the clinical departments plan and implement care with the input of residents and their loved ones.

PHYSICIAN SERVICES

Every nursing home is required to have physician services available as needed 7 days a week, 24 hours a day. These services are coordinated and supervised by the medical director (MD). Depending on the size of the facility, the MD may be part-time or full-time. Large facilities may also employ an assistant medical director.

Like other attending physicians who admit to the nursing home, the MD attends to a group of residents in the facility. In addition, the MD collaborates with the NHA and the director of nursing to establish policies and procedures for the facility. The MD also participates in facility committees, such as quality improvement.

Ideally the MD should be a geriatrician, a physician board certified in geriatric medicine. Many facilities are also seeking a physician who is certified as a medical director in long term care.

By federal law, each attending physician is obligated to make at least one visit every 60 days to each resident and document the resident's progress. As residents in nursing homes have become more acutely and chronically ill, many residents need more frequent physician visits. The nurse is responsible for communicating the resident's needs and progress to the attending physician. If the physician does not respond in a timely manner, the MD or assistant medical director is expected to handle the situation. Physicians who do not respond to the resident's needs, including the MD, can be fined by the state for noncompliance with state and federal regulations.

THE NURSING DEPARTMENT

The nursing department is the largest department within a nursing home. It is coordinated and managed by the director of nursing (DN or DON) and one or more assistant directors of nursing (ADNs or ADONs). If the nursing home is large enough, shift supervisors may also be used, especially for the evening and night shifts, or for the weekend when the DN and ADN are usually not in the building. These nurses are collectively referred to as nursing administration and are usually RNs.

As seen in Figure 11–1 (Chapter 11), each unit in the nursing home may have a unit coordinator (UC), nurse manager, or resident care coordinator who reports to the supervisor or ADN. The term used for this position varies from facility to facility. Smaller facilities may not have staff at this level in their organizational charts. The responsibility of the UC, typically an RN, is to coordinate and manage the unit, including managing staffing and resident issues.

Each nursing unit also has charge nurses who are "in charge" during each shift on the unit. The charge nurse, either an RN or LPN, makes resident assignments and oversees the operation of the unit during a particular shift. Under the charge nurse are other nurses and geriatric nursing assistants (or aides) (GNAs). A complete description of the charge nurse's responsibilities is found in Chapter 12.

The nursing care delivery system varies in each facility depending on the type and amount of staffing needed to meet resident acuity. On a traditional nursing unit, the number of GNAs is greater than the number of nurses. The GNAs are responsible for the majority of direct, routine resident care, including baths, changes of bed linen, feeding, transfers, and ambulation. Although staffing levels vary by facility, each GNA cares for an average of 8 to 10 residents during the day shift.

As mandated by federal law, GNAs must complete a course of study and take a national examination with both a written and clinical skills component. Then each GNA is registered with the state in which he or she is employed.

The nurses help the GNAs as needed but are primarily responsible for administering medications and performing prescribed treatments, including tube feedings. In addition to these nursing tasks and activities, nurses also use the nursing process to assess, plan, implement, and evaluate resident care. As discussed in Chapter 7, the nurse collaborates with other members of the health care team to develop and implement an interdisciplinary plan of care for each resident. The number of LPNs is usually greater than the number of RNs in most nursing homes because the resident population has a more stable health status than that found in acute care settings. Chapter 11 describes the structure and function of the nursing department in detail.

SOCIAL WORK DEPARTMENT

Every nursing home is required to have a social worker or a social work designee. The social worker should have a bacaalaureate degree in social work (BSW) as a minimum and preferably experience working in health care. A social work consultant with a master's degree may also be employed on a periodic basis to assist the social work staff. Social workers are usually licensed, by the state in which they are employed, on the basis of successfully completing an examination.

The primary responsibility of a social worker is to advocate for residents in a nursing home, ensuring that their rights as specified by federal and state law are not violated. The social worker also functions as a mediator between the resident's family, or significant others, and the facility.

He or she may also work with the local ombudsman to help resolve issues related to residents' rights. In collaboration with the nurse, the social worker typically plans for resident discharge.

DIETARY DEPARTMENT

The dietary department is responsible for preparing and distributing meals and snacks to the residents. It is usually coordinated by a food service manager who has had special training in meal preparation, sanitation, therapeutic diets, and employee management. The cooks prepare the meals, which are organized and delivered by the dietary aides.

Although a menu is prepared several weeks or months in advance, the dietary department must have alternate foods available for residents who dislike certain meals. Residents also have the right to eat when they wish, meaning that they can miss the hot breakfast and have a cold breakfast later if they desire. Most residents, however, chose to eat at the same time as the rest of the residents.

A registered dietitian (RD) collaborates with the department to plan menus and therapeutic diets to meet the special needs of some residents, such as those needing diabetic diets or sodium-restricted diets. In smaller nursing homes, the RD functions as a consultant and visits the facility anywhere from once a month to 1 or 2 days a week. Larger facilities may need a dietitian 3 days a week, or they may require a full-time dietitian as resident acuity level in the nursing home increases.

PHARMACY SERVICES

Few nursing homes have an in-house pharmacy. Therefore, an outside pharmacy in the community or a large pharmacy service delivers medications for use in the nursing home. Most facilities use a unit-dose system, in a 7-day or 30-day delivery system. The pharmacy delivers enough medications for a week or a month at a time, depending on nursing preference and cost considerations.

A back-up system, sometimes referred to as an "interim box," contains extra drugs that are commonly prescribed in the nursing home. This system allows residents to receive their medications promptly.

An emergency drug box or cabinet is also designated for drugs that must be given immediately as a resident's condition changes. For example, if a resident begins to develop congestive heart failure, a stat dose of furosemide (Lasix) and digoxin, as prescribed by the health care provider, can be administered without waiting for the drug to be delivered.

A consultant pharmacist is responsible for auditing the residents' charts. In this role, the pharmacist checks that doses are within the normal range and that the resident has not experienced untoward effects from drug therapy. He or she also ensures that the appropriate laboratory tests have been ordered as they are affected by drug therapy and looks for drug–drug or drug–food interactions. For example, a resident on diuretics needs frequent monitoring of serum electrolytes (at least monthly). A resident on phenytoin (Dilantin) needs at least a quarterly measurement of drug level to check for drug toxicity. Chapter 5 discusses drug therapy in more detail.

REHABILITATION SERVICES

Rehabilitation services include physical therapy, occupational therapy, and speech/language pathology, sometimes referred to as speech therapy. The collective goal of rehabilitation services is to assist the resident in returning to independent function, if possible, or to return to his or her baseline level of function. Rehabilitation programs for residents typically last from 4 to 6 weeks, but additional therapy may be needed in some cases.

Restorative therapy focuses on maintenance of function in activities of daily living (ADLs), including ambulation. Nursing, physical therapy, and occupational therapy work together in providing restorative care for residents.

Physical Therapy

The primary responsibility of the physical therapist is to help the resident become more mobile through therapeutic exercises, transfer training, and progressive ambulation, including the use of ambulatory aids, such as a walker or cane (Fig. 10–1). The therapist can also administer pain management techniques, such as heat, massage, and transelectric nerve stimulation applications.

The registered physical therapist (RPT) is an individual with a master's degree who has passed the state examination and has been licensed by the state. The RPT may have one or more physical therapy assistants (PTAs) who help the therapist with various activities. PTAs must be directly supervised by the registered physical therapist.

Occupational Therapy

The registered occupational therapist (OTR) is similar to a physical therapist in that he or she promotes resident independence in functioning, particularly in the ability to perform ADLs, which include feeding, bathing, dressing, grooming, and mobility. An occupational therapy assistant (OTA) may work with the OTR in implementing the rehabilitation

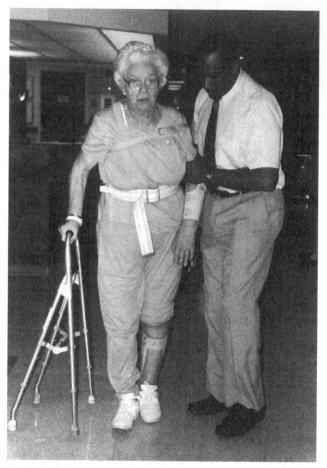

Figure 10–1. A physical therapist teaching a resident how to ambulate with a hemicane. Note that the cane is used on the strong side of the body.

program. OTAs must be directly supervised by the occupational therapist. A minimum of a baccalaureate degree and license are required for the OTR to practice.

Speech-Language Pathology

The speech-language pathologist (SLP) promotes independence by helping the resident gain speech and language skills. Among the elderly population, SLPs work most often with residents who have experienced speech and language deficits as a result of strokes. The SLP also specializes in evaluations of swallowing and in training for residents who have dysphagia, often those with strokes. She or he checks to see that diet consistency is appropriate for residents and sees that food texture is individualized as needed.

ACTIVITY THERAPY

In recent years, activity therapists have become essential members of the health care team in nursing homes. Unlike the OTR who plans therapeutic activities to regain ADL function, the activity therapist plans activities for recreational and therapeutic purposes. To the extent possible, the activities should be planned with resident input to determine what activities the residents enjoy. Activities should be planned for evenings and weekends, as well as during the day.

The activities should be geared to the cognitive level of the residents. For example, special activities should be planned for those residents with dementia. Activities must also be made available to bed bound residents.

Other activities should be tailored to younger residents. In some facilities, a young residents' support group meets on a regular basis and goes to movies, concerts, or other events that appeal to that age group. Out-of-facility activities are also arranged for older residents who are able to sit in a chair or wheelchair. Activity therapy assistants and GNAs are often needed to help the residents with these various activities.

Role of Nonclinical Departments

Several departments within a nursing home have no direct resident care responsibilities. Yet they are very important to the overall functioning of the facility.

ENVIRONMENTAL SERVICES

Environmental services is a newer term for the housekeeping department. The housekeepers generally work most often during the day (but some may have evening hours) and are responsible for cleaning the floors and residents' rooms. When a resident is discharged, the resident's unit (furniture and bed) must be disinfected before the next admission to the unit. Many of the housekeepers develop a close relationship with the residents and can be very helpful to the nursing staff in reporting unusual behaviors or preventing a fall.

LAUNDRY SERVICES

As the name implies, the laundry department washes and dries facility linens and the residents' personal clothing. Residents in a nursing home are encouraged to have their own clothing to help them feel more "at home." The families should be reminded to label all clothing and avoid expensive clothing that cannot hold up to commercial washers and dryers. Some facilities use outside contractors for laundry and other services. In this case, a washer and dryer are available if the resident wants to wash her or his own clothes.

MAINTENANCE DEPARTMENT

The maintenance department is responsible for ensuring that the physical plant remains in safe, working order and that the grounds of the facility remain safe and neat. The members of this department may also be asked to do minor renovations, remodeling, and general upkeep in areas within the facility.

STAFF DEVELOPMENT

In most nursing homes, a nurse is employed to provide staff development for the facility's employees. Federal and state regulations require that all staff have mandatory in-service programs on such topics as infection control, fire and safety, and residents' rights. GNAs are required by federal regulation to have additional mandatory hours of in-service education. In addition to providing these educational sessions, the staff development coordinator keeps records to show that the staff have attended the sessions.

The staff development coordinator may also provide or arrange for additional educational programs to keep the staff current in practice. The nursing home may have continuing education funds to assist employees in attending seminars that are held outside the facility.

For registered nurses, some of the outside programs may help meet requirements for certification as a gerontological nurse through the American Nurses Credentialing Center (ANCC). Gerontological nurse certification by the ANCC demonstrates that the nurse has specialized knowledge in the care of the elderly in a variety of settings. Table 10–1 lists the criteria for becoming certified.

CONTINUOUS QUALITY IMPROVEMENT

Also called quality assurance and total quality management, continuous quality improvement (CQI) is a process in which the nursing home reviews its care and compares it to preset standards for the industry. The program is organized and implemented by the CQI coordinator, who should involve all staff in every department. The CQI coordinator should report directly to the NHA because all departments are involved. However, in some facilities the coordinator reports to the DN. Some nursing homes rely on corporate staff for CQI activities. Chapter 14 describes CQI in detail.

Table 10–1. **Criteria for ANCC Gerontological Nurse Certification**

Licensed as a registered nurse*
Worked as a nurse in any role for 4000 hours
Worked as a nurse in any role over the past 2 years for 2000 hours; 51% of nursing care was for individuals over 65 years of age
Received 30 hours of continuing education (CE) over the past 2 years in the care of the elderly (20% can be obtained from written CE tests from journals)
Passed the gerontological nurse examination administered by the ANCC
Fulfilled criteria for recertification every 5 years (150 hours of CE credit, presentations, or publishing)

*Beginning in 1998, the nurse will need a baccalaureate in nursing degree to take the certification examination.
ANCC = American Nurses Credentialing Center

CENTRAL OFFICE STAFF

The central office staff usually includes a group of receptionists and secretaries who report to the office manager. These individuals provide clerical support for the NHA and other departments within the nursing home. The accounting and bookkeeping staff may work within the central office of the facility or may be located at a corporate office.

MEDICAL RECORDS CONSULTANT

Most nursing homes employ one or more consultants for areas that do not require full-time employment. For example, a registered records administrator (RRA) or registered records technician (RRT) may consult with the nursing home every quarter, or more often, to check on how the medical records are being kept. The consultant makes recommendations for improvement to the administrator as needed.

CHAPTER HIGHLIGHTS

Nursing home ownership may be for-profit, not-for-profit, nonprofit, or the home may be government operated.

The primary role of the nursing home administrator (NHA) is to ensure quality resident care in a cost-effective manner; the NHA is responsible for the day-to-day operation of the facility and reports to ownership.

The clinical departments provide direct, "hands-on" care to the residents; examples include physician services, rehabilitation services, nursing department, social work, and pharmacy services.

Rehabilitation services include physical therapy, occupational therapy, and speech and/or language pathology.

The nonclinical departments do not provide direct resident care but are important to the overall functioning of the facility.

Social work, dietitian, pharmacy, and medical records consultants are commonly used in the nursing home setting.

REFERENCES AND READINGS

Burke, M. M., & Walsh, M. B. (1997). *Gerontologic nursing: Wholistic care of the older adult* (2nd ed.). St. Louis: Mosby.
Matteson, M. A., McConnell, E. S., & Linton, A. D. (1997). *Gerontological nursing: Concepts and practice* (2nd ed.). Philadelphia: W. B. Saunders.
Ringsven, M. K., & Bond, D. (1997). *Gerontology and leadership skills for nurses* (2nd ed.). Albany, NY: Delmar.

DISCUSSION QUESTIONS TO PROMOTE CRITICAL THINKING

1. You are an RN working in a nursing home. One of your GNAs asks you why she needs to ambulate Mrs. Brown because that should be the physical therapist's job. What response would you give her?

2. One of the brakes on a resident's wheelchair does not function properly. What department in the nursing home should be called to repair it, and why?

3. The consultant pharmacist writes on a chart that a resident should not be given Haldol, a potent psychotropic drug, as prescribed because it is a chemical restraint. The resident has exhibited no behaviors that warrant this drug and is becoming increasingly sedated. As the charge nurse, what should you do in this situation?

11 Organization and Function of the Nursing Department

OBJECTIVES

- Describe the roles and responsibilities of the director of nursing in a nursing home
- List the qualifications for a director of nursing
- Describe the relationship of quality improvement, risk management, utilization review (utilization management), and infection control
- Identify three models for the delivery of nursing care: functional model, team nursing, and resident-focused care
- Differentiate the responsibilities of the geriatric nursing assistant/aide and certified medicine aide
- Identify the role of the case manager in long term care

The nursing department (ND) of a nursing home is typically the largest department within the organization. Unlike other departments, the nursing department provides staff for resident care every day, 24 hours a day. Although the sizes and types of nursing homes vary somewhat, most NDs are similar in organizational structure and function.

Historically, the nursing department was referred to as "nursing service." The term "service," however, seems to reinforce the subordinate role of nurses—an image that the profession has worked hard to overcome. The ND is headed by the director of nursing, who is sometimes called the nurse executive, nurse administrator, or similar title.

Director of Nursing

The typical organization of the nursing department in a nursing home is illustrated in Figure 11–1. As mentioned in the previous chapter, the upper-level positions of the department are collectively referred to as nursing administration. According to the Omnibus Budget Reconciliation Act (OBRA) of 1987, the ND of a skilled facility must be headed by a director of nursing (DN or DON) who is an RN and works full-time in the DN position. He or she coordinates and oversees the day-to-day operation of the nursing department.

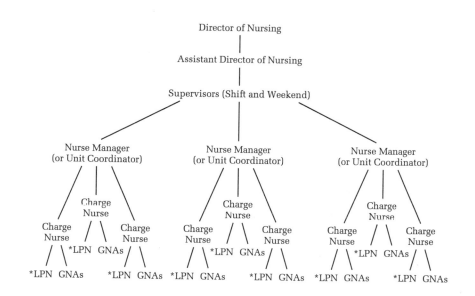

* LPN may not be needed. Charge nurse may be the only nurse on the unit.

Figure 11–1. Structure of a nursing department.

ROLES AND RESPONSIBILITIES OF THE DIRECTOR OF NURSING

Like the other department heads, the DN reports to the nursing home administrator and participates in department head meetings. As listed in Table 11–1, the DN has multiple responsibilities. In general, the DN is responsible for planning, organizing, managing, and evaluating the nursing department. Some of the major responsibilities are discussed in more detail below.

The National Association of Directors of Nursing Administration in Long Term Care (NADONA-LTC) provides an opportunity for DNs and assistant directors of nursing (ADNs) to network and participate in educational programs. Some states have local chapters as well. NADONA-LTC also offers a certification examination for DNs and ADNs.

Budget Preparation

One of the DN's primary responsibilities is monitoring the department's budget. Some nursing home administrators do not involve their department heads in the budget process. However, the DN should know best what the needs of the department are and, therefore, should have the responsibility of preparing, revising, and monitoring the budget as part of his or her responsibilties.

When preparing the budget, the DN should solicit input from the nursing staff regarding the needs of the department. If feasible, these needs may become part of the requested *operational* budget in which the facility's expenses and needs are balanced by the revenues (income) to the facility.

The staff or nursing administration may also request items for the *capital* budget. Put simply, the capital budget is reserved for larger or

Table 11–1. **Areas of Responsibility for the Director of Nursing in a Nursing Home**

Nursing department budget preparation
Nursing department budget monitoring
Staffing and monitoring of all units at appropriate levels
Recruitment and retention of nursing staff
Employee discipline and performance appraisals
Coordination of interdisciplinary resident care team
Quality improvement activities
Infection control
Risk management
Utilization review and management
Resident care studies
Resource for staff
Public relations and marketing to families and community at large

more expensive items that are "one time" purchases or costs. Examples of capital expenditures include bedscales, beds, wheelchairs, or the building of additional square footage for the facility. The capital budget does not rely solely on revenues to the facility. It may be funded by loans, investors, or donations. Therefore, the operational budget and capital budget must be kept separate. Funds from one budget should not be used for the other.

Clinical Programs

In smaller facilities, the DN may also be responsible for infection control, risk management, and quality improvement programs. In larger facilities, nurses or other health care professionals fill separate positions for each of these programs. Nursing homes that are part of large corporate structures also have the support of corporate staff who specialize in each of these program areas.

Infection control activities include tracking and monitoring infections, as well as implementing measures to prevent infection. An infection report may be initiated by a staff or charge nurse and submitted to the director of nursing. If outbreaks of influenza or other infections occur, the DN or other infection control designee may need to initiate strategies to prevent the spread of infection, such as a temporary ban on admissions to the facility, restriction of visitors, and the limiting of group resident activities. Most states also require that infection outbreaks be reported to the local or state health department.

Risk management is the term used for promoting resident safety and preventing medical malpractice throughout the facility. The primary tool that the DN or other designee uses to track potential safety or malpractice problems is the incident report. As described in Chapter 7, the incident report is usually completed by a nurse or other staff member and submitted to the DN. These data are summarized and analyzed to identify actual or potential problems related to resident care. Examples of resident care issues are falls and medication errors. Once a problem has been identified, an action plan is implemented and evaluated for its effectiveness in resolving the problem.

The DN oversees this process and reports findings to the nursing home administrator and the quality improvement (QI) committee. The QI committee, formerly called the quality assurance (QA) committee, is an interdisciplinary group of staff members who review data, help formulate action plans, and follow up on trends for actual or potential care issues.

A comprehensive QI program includes infection control, risk management, utilization review (UR) and management, and clinical studies. Utilization review and management is a process in which the level of care that a resident needs is periodically evaluated in collaboration with the health care team. For example, the UR committee (usually a subset of the QI committee) may determine that a resident no longer requires a skilled level of care because the resident has met his or her goals in a rehabilitation program. In this case, once the resident's level of care changes, Medicare is no longer the reimbursement source for payment. Medicare pays only for skilled care.

Clinical studies may result from risk management activities or from other identified resident concerns. An example of a clinical study is described later in this chapter under "Quality Improvement Coordinator."

QUALIFICATIONS OF THE DIRECTOR OF NURSING

Many DNs currently employed by nursing homes do not have a baccalaureate degree in nursing. However, in view of the tremendous responsibilities that accompany the position, there is a growing trend to employ nurses with a baccalaureate or master's degree.

The DN must be able to comprehend "the big picture," especially the financial aspects associated with long term care. Effective leadership and management skills, particularly the ability to communicate as part of an interdisciplinary team, are also essential.

Assistant Director of Nursing

Nursing homes with more than 100 beds usually have an assistant director of nursing. Extremely large facilities may have more than one ADN. As the name implies, the ADN assists the DN in meeting the goals of the nursing department and the facility. The DN delegates those tasks and activities which he or she feels can be successfuly accomplished by the ADN. In most facilities, a major role for the ADN is preparing work schedules and addressing staffing needs. The ADN may also represent the nursing department at weekly resident-care planning meetings. Both the ADN and DN may periodically substitute for the charge or staff nurses to meet special staffing needs.

Quality Improvement Coordinator

Part of the OBRA legislation enacted in 1990 was the requirement that a quality assessment and assurance (QAA) committee meet quarterly to identify and manage actual and potential problems related to resident care. Although the terms QAA or QA (quality assurance) may still be used by some facilities, the current trend is to replace them with quality improvement (QI), continuous quality improvement (CQI), or total quality management (TQM). *Assuring* quality is perhaps an unrealistic goal, but quality should improve over time.

The QI committee is an interdisciplinary group which reviews the results of clinical studies. Each department of the nursing home should conduct QI studies, selecting the high risk, high volume, high cost, problem-prone concerns. The facility may have a QI coordinator, usually a nurse, who reports to the DN or nursing home administrator. The coordinator may assist each department as they develop their QI program.

The QI process is very similar to the nursing process. A clinical area of concern is assessed and a goal (called an indicator or standard) is established. For instance, the nursing staff might be concerned about the incidence of facility-acquired pressure ulcers. A desired goal might be that less than 1 percent of all pressure ulcers will be acquired in the nursing home. Data collection during a 3-month monitoring period may show a total of 10 ulcers, but that only 2 developed in the facility. In this example, the incidence of facility-acquired pressure ulcers is 2 in 10 or 20 percent, well above the desired level.

The nursing department analyzes these data and develops an action plan to reduce the development of presssure ulcers. After the action plan is implemented, additional data to evaluate the success of the plan are needed. The data, plan, and results are reported to the QI committee. The process is ongoing, and the problem is readdressed as needed.

Nursing Supervisor

Large facilities usually employ shift supervisors, also known as "house supervisors," who represent nursing administration and oversee the nursing department on the evening, night, and weekend shifts. Nursing supervisors are typically RNs who are available as resources for the staff.

Minimum Data Set Coordinator

Since the requirement for completing a comprehensive assessment was initiated in 1990, many facilities have hired nurses to complete an assessment of every resident on admission and update the assessment as required. The federal assessment tool that all nursing homes use is the Minimum Data Set (MDS) described in Chapter 7. Additional assessment tools may be required, depending on the state. In the near future, the federal government will require that all MDS assessments be automated. The nurse responsible for this process is sometimes called the MDS coordinator.

Unit Coordinator

A unit coordinator (UC) is a middle management position usually held by an RN. Also called the unit director, nurse manager, or other title, the UC oversees the day-to-day operation of one or more units within the nursing home and has 24-hour responsibility for the unit. As the name implies, he or she coordinates the activities of the unit and supervises unit staff.

Charge Nurse

The charge nurse is the nurse who is responsible for resident care on a given unit in the nursing home. Typically, each shift has an identified charge nurse. Both RNs and LPNs/LVNs may hold the position of charge nurse. Chapter 12 discusses the role of the charge nurse in detail.

Staff Nurse

Nurses who report to the charge nurse are staff nurses, either RNs or LPNs/LVNs. Depending on the nursing care delivery system used in the facility, the job of the staff nurse may focus on a particular aspect of care, such as medication administration or treatments. Although this functional approach to resident care may divide nursing tasks and activities easily, nursing care can become fragmented with this method.

In some nursing homes, the staff nurse functions as a team leader with responsibility for assessments, medication administration, treatments, and overall care management. The team nursing approach prevents fragmentation of care and facilitates care coordination.

One of the newest models for nursing care delivery is resident-focused care or resident-centered care. In this model, a nurse pairs with an unlicensed staff member to provide total care to a group of residents. The nurse also collaborates with members of the interdisciplinary team to help the resident meet expected quality outcomes. This model is most appropriate for a subacute unit, where professional staffing ratios are higher than in the traditional nursing home.

Geriatric Nursing Assistant/Aide

In most nursing homes the bulk of the nursing staff is made up of unlicensed geriatric nursing assistants (GNAs). GNAs receive at least 75 hours of training, including both a classroom and clinical practicum portion.

The graduates of the training must pass a test and be registered with the state in which they are employed.

The GNA performs most of the direct care for residents, including baths, bedmaking, incontinence and skin care, and mobility and ambulation activities. The nurse is accountable for the performance of the GNA and other staff members whom he or she supervises.

Certified Medicine Aide

Only a few states have approved the certified medicine aide (CMA) position. The CMA is usually a GNA who has had at least one year of experience in a nursing home and successfully completes a state-approved course of study. The CMA can administer oral medications and selected topical medications. CMAs work under the supervision and guidance of the nurse.

Care/Case Manager

The newest role in the nursing home setting is the case manager. As described in Chapter 9, case management is a care delivery process in which a large number of high-risk residents are carefully monitored throughout their course of treatment. The goal of case management is the achievement of optimum quality and cost outcomes.

Case management is not practiced in all nursing homes and tends to be most useful in subacute and skilled units. Residents admitted to these units usually have short-term stays of from 1 to 3 weeks.

The case management process is guided by a care or case manager (CM), who is most often a registered nurse with a baccalaureate degree. The CM could also be a respiratory therapist, social worker, or other health professional, depending on the type of residents in the setting. The CM coordinates services and resources for the resident in collaboration with members of the health care team.

According to the recent standards published by the Case Management Society of America (1995), the roles of the CM include assessment, planning, advocacy, implementation, monitoring, and evaluation. Although these roles are not new to nurses, monitoring the financial aspects of care has not traditionally been a part of nursing education. The case manager must balance quality care with cost-effective care.

The CM may report directly to the unit coordinator or director of nursing. In very large facilities, a CM coordinator may oversee the activities of multiple case managers.

While the qualifications for a case manager in long term care have not been standardized, certain knowledge and competencies are essential. For

Table 11–2. **Knowledge and Competencies Needed for Care and/or Case Managers in Long Term Care**

- The aging process and differentiation from pathologic processes
- Chronic disease and acute illness management, especially in the elderly
- Special clinical problems such as falls, undernutrition, pressure ulcers
- Geriatric pharmacology
- Health promotion and illness prevention in the elderly and other populations
- Elder abuse and neglect, including reporting requirements and support agencies
- Legal aspects, including advance directives, competence issues
- Resolution of ethical dilemmas, such as cardiopulmonary resuscitation (CPR), tube feeding
- Community resources for discharge planning, including home care
- Continuum of services, such as assisted living, retirement centers
- Eligibility requirements for payer sources, such as Medicare, medical assistance, Veterans Administration, long term care insurance
- Americans with Disabilities legislation
- Quality of life issues
- Family dynamics and caregiver roles and needs
- Functional and cognitive assessments
- Development of a plan of care, including identified quality and cost outcomes
- Interdisciplinary communication and collaboration
- Negotiation and advocacy
- Leadership and management

example, the CM must have expert communication skills, including negotiation, advocacy, and collaboration. The CM works with external case managers employed by managed care organizations and traditional third-party payers to negotiate what care is needed at what cost for each resident. Long term care CMs must also understand the aging process and the common illnesses and diseases that affect the elderly. Table 11–2 lists important knowledge and skills that CMs need to effectively function in their role.

CHAPTER HIGHLIGHTS

The director of nursing (DN) in a nursing home is responsible for the overall operation of the nursing department, which may include budget preparation and monitoring, performance appraisals, and clinical programs.

A comprehensive quality improvement (QI) program encompasses infection control, risk management, utilization review and management, and resident care (clinical) studies.

A QI coordinator, who reports to the DN or nursing home administrator, may oversee the QI program.

The QI committee reviews and analyzes data, develops improvement plans, and evaluates whether the plans have been effective in resolving actual or potential resident care concerns.

The unit coordinator holds a middle management position and has 24-hour responsibility for an individual unit in a nursing home.

Nursing care may be delivered using the traditional functional nursing model, team nursing model, or the newer resident-focused model.

A certified medicine aide is a geriatric nursing assistant who has successfully completed a state-approved program to allow administration of oral and topical medications.

REFERENCES AND READINGS

Case Management Society of America (CMSA). (1995). *Standards for case management.* Little Rock, AR: Author.

Ringsven, M. K., & Bond, D. (1997). *Gerontology and leadership skills for nurses* (2nd ed.). Albany, NY: Delmar.

DISCUSSION QUESTIONS TO PROMOTE CRITICAL THINKING

1. The nursing staff of a local nursing home has complained that they are not getting a raise this year because the census of the facility has been lower than usual. One of your friends who is an LPN tells you that she thinks not getting more money is unfair because the owners are planning to build an addition to the building. How might you respond to her concern?

2. How might the staff working the 3–11 PM or 11 PM–7 AM shift utilize their nursing supervisor as a resource?

3. The role of the case manager in long term care is new but growing. Why do you think this position will be more popular in the future?

12 Role of the Charge Nurse

OBJECTIVES

- Define the term "charge nurse" as used in the nursing home setting
- Identify the major roles and responsibilities of the charge nurse
- Identify the relationship between delegation and supervision
- Briefly describe five strategies for conflict management
- Contrast three styles of leadership

The role of charge nurse is a traditional one, and nurses still fill this role in many nursing homes and hospitals. As the title implies, the charge nurse (CN) is a nurse who is "in charge" of the staff working on a resident care unit for a set period of time; the nurse is often referred to as the "7–3 shift charge nurse," the "3–11 charge nurse," and the "11–7 charge nurse."

Although the CN may be a registered nurse or a licensed practical (or vocational) nurse, LPNs often assume the role, especially in nursing homes. Some state boards of nursing are reexamining the use of LPNs as charge nurses to ensure that the LPN is not used in a position that needs the knowledge, skills, and abilities of an RN.

Staffing Patterns

While the charge nurse does not typically design the staffing pattern or schedule, he or she assesses the need for various levels of staff and shares this assessment with nursing administration. The traditional nursing home unit usually has 30 to 45 residents. For a unit of this size, a typical staffing pattern for the day shift (e.g., 7 AM to 3 PM) might include one nurse (who functions as the charge nurse) and four to six geriatric nursing assistants (GNAs). If the unit is designated as a skilled unit, a medicine aide (if sanctioned in the state) or second nurse may be added, depending on the acuity level of the residents. Subacute care units usually require higher staffing ratios, depending on the type of unit and the complexity of resident care. The budgeted hours of care per resident day determine the number of staff. Federal and state regulations delineate the minimum number of hours for each type of facility.

Most nursing homes reduce the number of staff on the evening and night shifts and during all weekend shifts. However, in the evening some elderly residents experience "sundowning" and become disoriented and confused. They are also fatigued from the day's activities and therefore may need as much staff and supervision as that provided by the day shift, if not more.

Roles and Responsibilities of the Charge Nurse

The charge nurse may provide clinical, hands-on resident care, such as medications, assessments, documentation, and treatments, discussed earlier in the book. In some facilities, the charge nurse provides less direct care and more supervisory activities. This section discusses the additional roles and responsibilities of the nurse who has the charge position.

SHIFT REPORT

The oncoming charge nurse and staff typically meet with the outgoing charge nurse to receive the shift report. However, in some facilities, the GNAs may not be included in the shift report; they obtain information about the residents directly from the oncoming nurse at the beginning of the shift. In other agencies, a taped report may be used rather than a face-to-face verbal report.

The shift report includes information about each resident's condition and concerns that need follow-up. Based on these data, the charge nurse can make a decision about staff assignments and priorities for resident care.

STAFF ASSIGNMENTS

One of the primary responsibilities of the CN is to organize and assign the staff for resident care. When assigning the tasks and activities related to resident care, the CN takes many elements into account, such as the complexity of resident care and abilities of each staff member (Hansten & Washburn, 1994). Table 12–1 includes a list of factors that must be considered in making staff assignments.

DELEGATION AND SUPERVISION

When the charge nurse makes staff assignments, he or she delegates nursing tasks and activities to licensed and unlicensed staff, especially GNAs. As defined by the National Council of State Boards of Nursing, delegation is transferring the responsibility of performing selected nursing tasks and activities in selected situations to a competent individual (Hansten & Washburn, 1994).

Many nurses are afraid to delegate because they fear losing their licenses or they do not trust the staff to whom they are supposed to delegate. Some nurses may also fear loss of control and prefer to do the tasks and activities themselves. Delegation can help nurses set priorities and allow them to spend time on those higher level skills that only nurses can perform, such as assessments, medication administration, and resident teaching.

The definition of delegation, accepted by all state boards of nursing, emphasizes the need for nurses to assess the competence of the staff to whom they delegate.

In most facilities, competencies are assessed by the staff development or education department before the employee begins working on the resident unit. However, competencies should also be assessed at least annually to assure *continued* competence. While the Joint Commission on Accreditation of Healthcare Organizations (JCAHO) requires annual competence assessments, state and federal long term care regulations typically do not specify a time frame requirement. Once an employee is determined

---

Table 12–1. **Factors to Consider When Making Staff Assignments**

Competencies of the staff member
Role and scope of practice of the staff member
Nature and complexity of the task
Acuity level of the resident
Time in which the task needs to be done
Location of the resident
Preferred method or procedure for the task or activity
Rationale for the task or activity

to be competent, the documentation of specific skills that he or she can perform should be available to the charge nurse.

The CN also has the responsibility to supervise delegates by providing initial direction, guidance, and periodic inspection of employees while performing the delegated tasks. The amount of guidance and how often to observe the delegate is determined by the charge nurse based on his or her professional judgment.

TEAM BUILDING AND COMMUNICATION

A team is a group of people who work toward a common goal. In health care, team members collaborate to meet the goal of quality care at a reasonable cost. To strengthen the team-building process, members must communicate continuously.

Communication is a two-way process in which a sender provides a message that is perceived by the receiver. Effective communication involves at least two people who affect each other. Too often health team members assume that if they have given a message to a coworker, the message has been understood and perceived in the manner in which it was intended. Unfortunately, listening is not a strongly developed skill in most people, so that the meaning of a message can be distorted and misunderstandings arise.

Additionally, a number of variables affect the communication process. An individual's culture, education level, past experience, sensory abilities (e.g., visual and hearing acuity), and personality all affect how that individual sends or perceives the message. For example, nursing assistants in nursing homes may complain that they observe nurses sitting in the nurses' station rather than helping them with the physical labor associated with total resident care. In many cases, the GNAs are not aware of the nursing requirements for documentation in nursing homes. When nurses communicate this information, the GNAs are more knowledgable and thus more likely to function as team members.

Verbal face-to-face communication is usually more effective than written communication, including the "high tech" e-mail. As much as 90 percent of any message is communicated nonverbally. A face-to-face interaction allows the receiver to interpret the content as well as the intent of the message. It also allows the sender to reinforce the content of the message with facial expressions and hand gestures and to respond immediately to the perceptions or questions posed by the receiver. For instance, a posted memo stating a new policy about the staff's dinner schedule may be ignored if there is no explanation as to why the schedule was changed. However, if staff members are given a rationale for the change in dinner scheduling, they have the opportunity to discuss their feelings and receive answers to any questions about the new policy. This face-to-face interaction is more likely to result in compliance with the new policy. This example also points out the nature of change. People generally do not like change. They are comfortable with the status quo and are fearful or anxious about the unknown. Yet change can be very positive, particularly when it improves resident care.

The best way to implement change is to use a planned change process. The charge nurse or other "change agent" presents or summarizes the need for change and encourages input by the staff who will be affected by the change. The staff may need additional information about the need and rationale for change. Then a solution is selected and implemented with staff input. All staff members need encouragement and support during the implementation phase. Once they are comfortable with the change, it becomes incorporated into the facility's policies. For example, a 7 AM–3PM shift charge nurse of a resident care unit has data that support the need for increased ambulation of residents. The GNAs complain that they do not have time to ambulate residents because they are too busy with the total care residents who are bed-chair confined. The result is that ambulatory residents sit for long periods of time and lose muscle strength and mobility.

In such a situation, the charge nurse could choose to remind everyone about the need for routine assistance with ambulation. Even if the GNAs agree that residents need to be ambulated, though, they may still complain that their resident load is too heavy to provide the necessary assistance. A solution to this common problem is to use a restorative aide, provided by the nursing department. A GNA could be trained by the physical therapist in techniques for ambulation, assistive devices, transfers, and range-of-motion exercises. This restorative aide could spend the entire shift performing these activities, thus giving the regular aides more time to spend with the total care residents. The restorative aide may work 9 AM to 5 PM instead of 7 AM to 3 PM because most residents are typically not out of bed by 7 AM. The specific scheduling and job description of the aide could be decided by the staff with the charge nurse's guidance. Once the change is tried, the charge nurse and nursing administration must support the staff until their group effectiveness in resolving the problem can be evaluated.

CONFLICT MANAGEMENT

Creating change typically results in conflict. Such conflict is inevitable because everyone responds to change differently. Conflicts may not always have resolutions, but they can be managed.

Five strategies for conflict management are commonly used, although some methods are preferred over others. People often use *avoidance* as a coping mechanism when conflict occurs. Although avoidance is an easy strategy to employ, it is the least preferred method for managing conflict. In a study of nurses employed at three hospitals, Fowler et al. (1993)

found that nurses use withdrawal, or avoidance, as the most common strategy for dealing with conflict. When conflicts are avoided, they tend to get bigger; they seldom disappear.

The second method for managing conflicts is *competition*. Competition is an "I win, you lose" strategy in which self-interest predominates and others' interests are not considered. This method is sometimes used by physicians in physician–nurse relationship.

The opposite of competition is *accommodation*. When using accommodation, an individual considers others' interests over self-interest. This method may be useful when the conflictual situation is not important to the individual but should not be used routinely as a way to manage conflict. Many nurses use accommodation because they have low self-esteem and are not assertive enough to communicate their needs or opinions.

The fourth strategy for conflict management is *compromise*. This method is an "I win some and lose some, you win some and lose some" situation. While this strategy is not ideal, it may help to manage very complex conflicts.

Collaboration is a "win-win," time-consuming strategy that should be reserved for highly emotional, complex conflicts. The two or more parties involved in the conflict collaborate in the problem-solving process. Changing care delivery systems requires collaboration for successful implementation.

LEADERSHIP STYLES

The charge nurse is a manager of the unit for a specified period of time, as well as a leader. Leadership implies the ability to influence others. To be an effective leader, the nurse must be able to garner support from the staff while guiding them in the delivery of resident care.

Several leadership and management styles have been described in the literature, including autocratic, laissez-faire, and democratic styles. An *autocratic* leader is one who makes decisions without input from the followers. He or she dictates what has to be done, and the staff is expected to adhere to these expectations. In a crisis situation, an autocratic style may be useful.

A *laissez-faire* leader is one who allows events and situations to occur without any direction. This "hands-off" approach provides no real leadership, and followers (staff) have no guidance or support. However, this style of leadership may be very appropriate for highly motivated and skilled employees.

The ideal type of leader is one who solicits input and feedback from followers and then jointly, with the staff, finds solutions to problems. This *democratic* style of leadership is more time-consuming than the other styles but is more likely to be effective.

At times, democratic leaders have to make solo decisions when limitations of time or resources make it necessary. For example, in the case of an emergency, such as a fire or other disaster, the responsible charge nurse assigns the staff actions that he or she feels are needed in the situation. Staff input is not practical in an emergency.

EMPLOYEE PERFORMANCE

In most long term care facilities, the charge nurse does not hire or terminate employees (called associates in some settings). However, charge nurses should have input regarding who the staff on the unit will be.

For professional staff, licenses must be validated by the appropriate state board. Unfortunately, some individuals have fake licenses or licenses that have been suspended or revoked. Professional and personal references should also be checked. These activities are usually performed by the director or assistant director of nursing or by human resources personnel, if they are available.

Most employees are placed on a brief probationary period, usually 90 days, during which the employee's performance is evaluated. The person supervising the employee should be the one who evaluates his or her performance. The personnel policy manual outlines those infractions for which the employee needs counseling, disciplining, or termination.

The charge nurse may complete a performance appraisal at the end of the probationary period and at periodic intervals, such as every 6 to 12 months. The *performance appraisal* form, sometimes called an evaluation form, should parallel the employee's job description. In other words, employees should be evaluated on how well they perform their jobs, rather than on whether or not they wore their uniforms or were cheerful during their work.

The appraisal should also contain an area where weaknesses can be identified. For each weakness, mutual goals and target dates for improvement are mutually agreed upon.

Performance appraisals should not be unexpected or a surprise to the employee. The supervisor provides formal and informal feedback to employees between evaluation intervals. Formal feedback may include counseling or disciplinary action with documentation. A minor infraction, such as being tardy, may require a counseling session without specific disciplinary action. Figure 12–1 shows a sample counseling form with supporting documentation. More serious infractions, such as resident neglect, may result in suspension or even termination. All counseling and disciplinary actions should be recorded and supported with specific documentation. The charge nurse needs to be very familiar with the personnel policy manual and the labor laws that apply at the state and federal levels.

HAPPY HILLS NURSING HOME

EMPLOYEE COUNSELING RECORD

Name of employee: *Stephanie Jones*   Date: *4-17-97*

Description of the situation: *Stephanie has been more than 20 minute late three times this week. She states that her ride is often late and she doesn't own a car.*

Action plan with target date: *Stephanie has agreed to ask her cousin to take her to work or find someone else. She will let me know by 4-19-97 what her new arrangements for transportation are. We will follow-up on progress at the end of next week.*

Signature of Counselor: *Marlene Smith, CNC*

Signature of Employee: *Stephanie Jones*

Follow-up: _____

Figure 12–1. Sample of an employee counseling form.

CHAPTER HIGHLIGHTS

The charge nurse is one who is "in charge" of the nursing staff working on a resident unit for a set period of time, such as the 7 AM–3 PM shift.

The major roles and responsibilities of the charge nurse include shift report and coordination, staff assignments, supervision of staff, team building, and communication within the department and with other departments.

Delegation is the process in which the nurse transfers the authority to perform selected nursing tasks and activities to a competent individual.

Supervision is the process in which the nurse provides initial direction, guidance, and follow-up to staff members to whom nursing tasks have been delegated.

The charge nurse often acts as an agent for planning and implementing necessary changes.

Five strategies for conflict management are avoidance, competition, accommodation, compromise, and collaboration.

Three common styles of leadership are autocratic, laissez-faire, and democratic.

REFERENCES AND READINGS

Ellis, J. R., & Hartley, C. L. (1995). *Managing and coordinating nursing care* (2nd ed.). Philadelphia: J. B. Lippincott.

Fowler, A. R., Jr. et al. (1993). *Health Progress, 74*(5), 25–29.

Hansten, R. I., & Washburn, M. J. (1994). *Clinical delegation skills: A handbook for nurses.* Gaithersburg, MD: Aspen.

Huber, D. (1996). *Leadership and nursing care management.* Philadelphia: W. B. Saunders.

Tappen, R. M. (1995). *Nursing leadership and management: Concepts and practice.* Philadelphia: F. A. Davis.

DISCUSSION QUESTIONS TO PROMOTE CRITICAL THINKING

1. As a charge nurse on a 28-bed unit, you find that there are only two aides assigned this evening, instead of the usual three aides. How could you handle this situation?

2. At the end of your shift you discover that Mrs. Peters has not received her range-of-motion exercises as requested. The aide has left the unit for the day. What should you do?

3. Some nurses are afraid to delegate because they feel their licenses are "on the line." How would you respond to this concern?

13 The Survey Process

OUTLINE

The Survey Team
Survey Preparation
Entrance Conference and Orientation Tour
Resident Sampling
Quality Assessments
Information Analysis and Decision Making
Exit Conference
Follow-up Surveys
Voluntary Accreditation
Role of the Nurse

OBJECTIVES

- State the purpose of the standard survey process
- Describe the focus of the environmental quality assessment, the quality of care assessment, and the quality of life assessment
- State the function of the resident and family councils
- Identify the components of the drug therapy review
- Describe the purpose of the exit conference
- Differentiate between the accreditation process of the Joint Commission of Accreditation of Healthcare Organizations and the survey process
- Briefly identify the role of the nurse related to the survey or accreditation process

L ong term care (LTC) facilities—skilled nursing facilities (SNFs) and nursing facilities (NFs)—must follow numerous state and federal regulations. Failure to comply with these laws can result in deficiency citations, monetary fines, and/or loss of licensure or certification. Each facility is inspected by a survey team every 12 to 18 months, depending upon state practice. This review process is referred to as the *standard* survey.

The Survey Team

Each state employs its own surveyors and conducts its own survey process for facilities operating within its jurisdiction. While the process varies slightly from state to state, most survey teams consist of nurses, dietitians, and/or sanitarians. Team visits to each facility are unannounced. A team of three or four surveyors usually spends 3 to 4 days reviewing a single facility, the time depending on the size and case mix within the nursing home.

The survey team follows a structured, predetermined process and documents its findings from the visit. These findings become part of public record and, by federal law under the Omnibus Budget Reconciliation Act of 1987 (OBRA), must be posted in the facility in an area accessible to anyone who wants to review them. A discussion of the steps of the survey process listed in Table 13–1 follows.

Survey Preparation

Before the survey team arrives at a LTC facility, its members review records of previous survey visits. Each state maintains records on every

Table 13–1. **Steps of the Standard State Survey Process**

Survey preparation
Entrance conference
Orientation tour
Resident sampling
Quality assessments
- Environmental quality assessment
- Quality of care assessment
  - Drug therapy review
  - Dining room observation
  - Closed record review
  - Dietary services system assessment
  - Medication pass
- Quality of life assessment
Information analysis and decision making
Exit conference
Follow-up survey (if needed)

facility it surveys. A recently developed scoring system rates each facility based on a 3-year survey history. This "report card" reflects the quality of the facility and the care it has provided.

The team also reviews the fire marshal's report and contacts the local or state ombudsman to inform him or her of the impending survey visit. The ombudsman, an advocate for nursing home residents, informs the surveyors whether complaints have been received about the facility, the nature of the complaints, whether the complaints were validated, and whether there are complaints pending investigation. The ombudsman is also usually invited to participate in the exit conference at the end of the survey.

The facility prepares for the survey by completing forms that list the names and conditions of the residents. Many nursing homes conduct mock surveys to identify any problem areas before the state survey visit.

Entrance Conference and Orientation Tour

When the survey team members arrive at the nursing home, they meet with the administrator and discuss plans for the visit. Then they post signs announcing that the team is conducting a facility inspection and that team members are available to meet with residents privately.

The next step is the orientation tour, which is designed to:

- Provide an overview of the facility for the surveyors
- Introduce surveyors to residents and staff
- Identify possible patterns of poor care that can be investigated during the quality of care (QOC) assessment
- Identify interviewable residents who can participate in the residents' rights and QOC assessments
- Identify residents who are not interviewable to participate in the QOC assessment

During the tour, the surveyors pay special attention to quality of care, quality of life, and residents' rights problems, such as:

- Clinical signs and symptoms, for example, edema and contractures
- Resident grooming and dress
- Functional risk factors, including poor positioning and use of physical restraints
- Infection control
- Staff-resident interactions related to residents' privacy, dignity, and care needs, including staff response to residents' requests for assistance

Resident Sampling

The survey team selects a representative sample of residents to review during the visit. The sample is a mix of interviewable, noninterviewable, light care, and heavy care residents. The number of residents in the sample depends upon the size of the facility. In general, the larger the facility, the larger the sample will be.

Additional residents may be added to the sample if specialized rehabilitation is provided or special treatments such as suctioning and tracheostomy care are performed.

Quality Assessments

The quality assessments step is divided into three general areas:
1. Environmental quality assessment
2. Quality of care assessment
3. Quality of life assessment

ENVIRONMENTAL QUALITY ASSESSMENT

The primary purpose of the environmental quality assessment is to observe physical aspects in the facility's environment that affect residents' quality of life, health, and safety. During this step, the surveyors usually review all activity areas, all therapy areas, all common areas (resident lounges and hallways, storage areas), the emergency power supply, and water availability. In addition, several residents' rooms on each wing of the facility are inspected.

During this portion of the overall quality assessment, the surveyors usually observe the response of the staff to resident call lights. They also inspect the facility for its ability to create a "homelike" environment. Personal items and pictures should be visible in each resident's room.

QUALITY OF CARE ASSESSMENT

The general purpose of the QOC assessment is to determine whether the care provided by the facility has enabled residents to reach or maintain their "highest practicable physical, mental, and psychosocial well-being" (Department of Health and Human Services, 1992, p. 15). The surveyors assess QOC by comparing the resident's care plan to the actual condition of each resident.

For all residents in the selected sample, care provided by the staff and outcomes of that care are assessed. Table 13–2 lists the care areas that the surveyors commonly target.

Table 13–2. **Care Areas Reviewed as Part of the Quality of Care Assessment**

- Maintaining safety
- Preventing pressure ulcers
- Maintaining vision and hearing abilities
- Maintaining or improving functional ability (activities of daily living) and mobility
- Maintaining and improving psychosocial status, including social services and activities assessment and care planning
- Maintaining mental status
- Maintaining urinary continence or effectively managing incontinence
- Preventing abuse or neglect
- Reducing the use of physical and chemical restraints
- Maintaining or improving nutritional status and hydration
- Preventing and managing infectious diseases

The surveyors review the medical record of each sampled resident, including the Minimum Data Set (MDS), Resident Assessment Protocols (RAPs) summary sheet, and comprehensive interdisciplinary care plan. Then they validate information from the record by observing each resident during treatments and at various other times of the day over the entire survey period. Interviews of residents, family members, visitors, and staff may be conducted to collect more information and to verify and validate previously collected information.

The survey team uses additional steps to determine QOC, including a drug therapy review, dining observation review, closed record review, dietary services system assessment, and medication pass.

Drug Therapy Review

The drug regimen ordered by the health care provider (physician, nurse practitioner, or physician assistant) is carefully scrutinized by the survey team. Each drug order must be accompanied by the rationale for the drug's use; for example, "digoxin 0.125 mg for atrial fibrillation." The surveyors identify or question the use of unnecessary drugs, especially antipsychotic drugs.

Appropriate laboratory studies should also be ordered for residents receiving certain types of drugs. For instance, residents receiving medications that require a therapeutic serum level, such as theophylline preparations, digoxin, and lithium, need regular laboratory assessment to ensure that therapeutic levels are achieved. Other drugs, such as warfarin (Coumadin) and Synthroid, require periodic laboratory tests to evaluate their effectiveness; in these cases, coagulation studies and thyroid function studies, respectively.

If the results of laboratory testing are abnormal, the facility is obligated to contact the health care provider. The action taken or not taken must be documented in the medical record.

Dining Room Observation

The dining room observation review allows the survey team an opportunity to observe the quality of life and quality of care associated with the dining experience for residents in the sample—especially those on special diets, those with nutritional deficiencies, and those with pressure ulcers. At least eight residents in different dining areas are typically observed during two meals. The food served should conform to the planned daily menu and the type of diet ordered by the health care provider.

Closed Record Review

In addition to the medical record review of the sampled residents, several closed records are reviewed to examine the appropriateness and quality of care that the staff provided prior to a resident's transfer, discharge, or death. The surveyors review at least five closed records of residents transferred or discharged for the 3 to 6 months prior to the survey.

Dietary Services System Assessment

The surveyors focus on several areas as they assess the facility's dietary services. These include sanitation, adequacy of food preparation and delivery, and the quality of care associated with dining, such as food choices. The kitchen staff are observed preparing at least one meal. One of the surveyors also checks food temperatures, especially for potentially hazardous foods such as poultry. Food from selected diets (such as pureed or low salt) may be tasted for palatability.

Medication Pass

One or more surveyors assess the preparation and administration of medications to detect errors. Two or more nurses or certified medicine aides (if state approved) are observed and the facility's medication error rate is computed. Appendix F lists the operational standards for the medication pass.

QUALITY OF LIFE ASSESSMENT

The purpose of the quality of life (QOL) assessment, also called the residents' rights assessment, is to determine how the facility protects and promotes residents' rights and enhances the quality of life for each resident. The survey team interviews individual residents, groups of residents, and residents' family members.

The surveyors usually ask the resident council if they can attend one of their meetings or a special meeting for the interview. In general, the

Table 13-3. Residents' Rights Areas Reviewed as Part of the Quality of Life Assessment

- Telephone and mail services
- Daily routines and activities
- Meals and snacks
- Roommates and room arrangements
- Personal money matters
- Contact with health care providers
- Resident involvement in decisions about care and treatment
- Safety and personal property considerations
- Privacy and dignity
- Complaints

purpose of this group is to discuss issues related to resident care and the operation of the facility. In facilities that also have a family council, the surveyors may ask this group for an interview as well. The family council consists of family members or significant others and also discusses issues related to care and the operation of the facility. Table 13-3 lists areas the surveyors typically target for the QOL assessment.

Information Analysis and Decision Making

After all the data have been collected, the survey team must review and analyze the data to determine whether the facility is in compliance with the regulatory requirements and whether to extend the standard survey for a more thorough review and analysis (called an *extended* survey). Areas in which the facility is *not* in compliance are identified and recorded as *deficiencies*. Depending on the severity of the deficiency (ies), a facility may be fined or have an extended survey. In cases of *severe* noncompliance, an SNF may lose its Medicare and Medicaid certification status and/or its license to operate as a long term care facility. An NF may lose its Medicaid certification and/or its license as well.

Exit Conference

The survey team informs the facility of its observations and findings at the exit conference. Facility staff, the ombudsman, and an officer of the resident council may attend. Specific references to residents are kept confidential by referring to the residents' number. A copy of the surveyors' report is left with the administrator, who is responsible for developing a plan of correction and submitting the plan to the state within a given time frame, usually 15 to 20 days after the survey or after the state decides on the level (severity) of the deficiency.

Follow-up Surveys

If the facility received any deficiencies and a plan of correction was filed, the survey team may return to the facility to ensure that the plan was implemented and improvements were made. The follow-up survey is usually a 1- to 2-day visit, depending on the number of deficiencies that need follow-up.

Voluntary Accreditation

In addition to the state survey, a facility may choose to become accredited through a voluntary accreditation process, such as that provided by the Joint Commission on Accreditation of Healthcare Organizations (JCAHO). In a few states, an LTC facility may select the JCAHO accreditation process *instead of* the state survey process to determine compliance with state and federal regulations. This alternative to the state process is expected to become more widely available as state and federal funding dwindles and governments seek new ways to save money.

For a JCAHO review, the facility pays a team of surveyors to inspect the facility for compliance with JCAHO requirements. The advantage of this additional recognition is the ability to apply for certain grants and funding, as well as the ability to train medical students, interns, and medical residents. Additionally, the inspection is announced and is felt by many facilities to be more helpful than the state survey process. Chapter 9 discusses JCAHO accreditation and other voluntary accreditations for subacute care units.

Role of the Nurse

All nurses working in nursing homes need to be very knowledgeable about the federal and state regulations governing the operation of nursing homes. If the facility is seeking JCAHO accreditation, nurses need to become familiar with the standards that JCAHO publishes for long term care and to share this information with unlicensed staff.

Another major responsibility for nurses is to maintain thorough, accurate documentation, including the MDS and comprehensive care plan. Chapter 7 contains a detailed discussion of documentation in the long term care setting.

CHAPTER HIGHLIGHTS

The purpose of the standard state survey process is to determine if long term care (LTC) facilities are in compliance with state and federal regulations.

The focus of the environmental quality assessment step of the survey process is observation of the physical aspects in the facility's environment that affect residents' quality of life, health, and safety.

The general purpose of the quality of care assessment is to determine whether the care provided by the facility has enabled residents to reach or maintain their "highest practicable physical, mental, and psychosocial well-being."

The primary focus of the quality of life assessment is the determination of how the facility protects and promotes residents' rights and the quality of life for each resident.

The purpose of the resident and family councils is to provide a forum for discussion of resident care issues and facility operation.

The survey team informs the facility of its observations and findings at the exit conference.

In most states, the state survey process is mandatory; the accreditation process of the Joint Commission on Accreditation of Healthcare Organizations is voluntary.

Nurses in LTC facilities must know the state and federal regulations and the importance of accurate and complete documentation in the medical record; the surveyors rely on the medical record to assist them with the survey process.

REFERENCES AND READINGS

Department of Health and Human Services, Health Care Financing Administration (Pub. 7). (1992). *State Operations Manual.* Springfield, VA: U.S. Department of Commerce, National Technical Information Service.

DISCUSSION QUESTIONS TO PROMOTE CRITICAL THINKING

1. Does a resident have the right to mail letters listing complaints about a nursing home that have not been validated? Why or why not?

2. What suggestions do you have to address residents' concerns about a facility's food?

3. The nursing home where you work was cited by the surveyors for errors in transcription of physician's orders, particularly medication dosages. How could this deficiency be corrected? Write a realistic plan of correction.

14 The Quality Improvement Process

OUTLINE

Quality Assurance and Assessment
Total Quality Management
Statistical Analysis
Staff Feedback

OBJECTIVES

- Define the terms quality assessment, quality assurance, total quality management, and continuous quality improvement
- Differentiate three types of standards: structure, process, and outcome standards
- Describe the relationship between total quality management, continuous quality improvement, risk management, performance management, and utilization review (utilization management)

Quality is a difficult concept to define. In general, quality is related to standards of excellence. Health care agencies of all types strive to provide the highest quality of care possible.

Before the enactment of the Omnibus Budget Reconciliation Act (OBRA) of 1987, long term care (LTC) facilities were not required to have an organizational program that examined their ability to provide quality care. In essence, the annual state survey inspection served this purpose by citing aspects of care in which facilities were deficient (see Chapter 13).

The 1987 OBRA legislation mandated the establishment of an interdisciplinary quality assessment and assurance (QAA) committee, which must meet at least quarterly. Beyond this requirement, LTC facilities choose the extent to which care is reviewed and improved.

Quality Assurance and Assessment

Quality assurance (QA) refers to a facility's ability to provide health care services according to professional and regulatory standards. QA builds on quality assessment, which is the measurement of quality. The QA approach takes statistical data about resident care from the quality assessment, analyzes the data, and takes action to improve care if needed.

STANDARDS

Standards define quality; therefore, resident care is measured against predetermined standards. Standards come from a variety of sources, including federal and state laws, the American Nurses Association, and policies and procedures set forth by the facility. Donabedian (1980) developed one of the earlier frameworks for standards. He stated that quality can be measured using structure, process, and outcome standards.

Structure Standards

Structure standards focus on the resources and internal characteristics of the facility, such as the physical plant, staffing, financial resources, and formal policies and procedures. This group of standards examines whether or not the facility has adequate structure in place to promote quality care. An example of a structure standard might be: The supply budget is adequate to meet the needs of the residents.

Process Standards

Process standards focus on the actual tasks and activities involved in providing care. This group of standards examines whether or not the staff is performing at the expected level. An example of a process standard might be: The RN will perform an initial resident assessment within 24 hours of admission.

Outcome Standards

Perhaps the most measurable and most important type of standard is the outcome standard. Outcomes refer to the result of care provided for the residents, including the residents' physical health status, mental health status, social function, health care knowledge, and perceptions of the level of care provided. An example of an outcome standard might be: The resident will have intact skin that is clean and dry.

AUDITS

One method for evaluating whether or not identified standards have been met is to conduct audits to measure indicators of quality. An indicator is an objective, measurable variable of care, such as infection rate, incidence of falls, and medication errors. An audit, typically a chart audit, is one of the most common methods for quality assessment. In this technique, data are collected from various charts to determine if standards were met. Nursing audits can be grouped into three types: prospective, concurrent, and retrospective audits.

Prospective audits are done *before* care occurs. Potential problems are identified, such as risk for falls or pressure ulcers, and programs to prevent these problems are implemented. Concurrent audits are done *during* care. Documenting variances from a predetermined plan of care is an example of a concurrent audit. Retrospective audits are done *after* care is provided. These audits allow evaluation of resident outcomes to determine if the desired expected outcomes were achieved.

Total Quality Management

Although it is still sometimes used, the term *quality assurance* is outdated, because it focuses only on clinical standards and outcomes of care. The most current concepts are called total quality management (TQM) and continuous quality improvement (CQI). Although sometimes used interchangably, these terms are somewhat different. TQM is a structured, organization-wide program that serves as an umbrella for the CQI, risk management, performance management, and utilization review/management processes (Fig. 14–1).

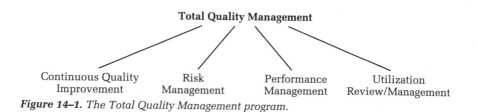

Figure 14–1. *The Total Quality Management program.*

CONTINUOUS QUALITY IMPROVEMENT

Continuous quality improvement is the comprehensive process of continuously evaluating and improving health care services, and it involves all departments in an agency or facility. All levels of staff should be involved in the process. For instance, nursing assistants observe residents' skin for intactness and cleanliness and can record these observations.

CQI addresses outcomes of care, including clinical outcomes, cost outcomes, and customer satisfaction. Customers are residents, staff, families and/or significant others, health care professionals, and the community.

A variety of assessment tools are used to continuously evaluate and monitor quality, including audits, observation, checklists, rating scales, questionnaires, and time-and-motion studies (Huber, 1996). For example, the use of resident satisfaction surveys is a method of evaluating each resident's and family's satisfaction with the care provided by the facility.

The nursing home may employ an individual called a QA or CQI coordinator to organize and oversee the CQI program. Because CQI is an organization-wide process, the QA or CQI coordinator is most often a nurse who reports to the nursing home administrator. In some facilities, the nursing home administrator or director of nursing may be responsible for CQI activities.

RISK MANAGEMENT

Risk management (RM) includes, but is not limited to, prevention and monitoring of accidents, incidents, malpractice, and a wide variety of legal issues. RM may be coordinated by an individual in the organization called a risk manager. The director of nursing, nursing home administrator, or CQI coordinator may assume this role in small, independent facilities.

The function of the risk manager is to implement systems that prevent and monitor situations placing the facility at risk for legal action or poor customer relations. For example, some facilities have a safety committee to inspect the physical plant for hazards or potential hazards. These concerns are recorded and shared with the administrator and the appropriate departments affected by their findings.

The risk manager also reviews and analyzes all incident reports. Sometimes called unusual occurrence or variance reports, incident reports provide a record of information regarding events that could potentially increase the facility's liability. The risk manager or designee reviews the reports, analyzes them, and draws conclusions about actual or potential problems. These problems are shared with department heads and the TQM/CQI committee, where an action plan to correct each problem is developed and readied for implementation. After a specified period of time, data from incident reports are collected, reviewed, and analyzed to determine if the action plan was successful in solving the problem. Table 14–1 summarizes an example of this process.

PERFORMANCE MANAGEMENT

Performance management is a program that looks at employee performance in meeting expectations and standards for the facility. It measures quality on an individual level by comparing employee function with facility expectations as outlined in the job or role description. For employees who do not meet job expectations, a performance improvement plan should be developed to help them reach the expected level of performance.

A performance appraisal, sometimes referred to as an employee evaluation, is a document that summarizes the employee's performance at regular intervals, often annually. Employees should be evaluated on their performance rather than their personalities, friendliness, appearance, and so forth. Many evaluation tools assess these areas instead of focusing on the actual performance of the employee. The crucial question is: How well did the employee perform his or her job?

UTILIZATION REVIEW (UTILIZATION MANAGEMENT)

Utilization review (UR) was originally mandated by the federal government as part of quality monitoring for Medicare reimbursement. The

Table 14–1. **Summary of Study on Resident Falls**

- Data collected from incident reports over 6 months:
  - Average of one fall per day
  - 70% of falls occur between 4 PM and 8 PM
  - Average age of residents who fall is 82
  - 80% of falls occur in resident rooms
- Factors possibly contributing to falls between 4 PM and 8 PM:
  - Smaller number of nursing staff on 3–11 PM shift
  - Fewer members of the administrative, maintenance, social work, and housekeeping staff in the facility
  - Residents fatigued and "sundowning" from day's activities
  - Residents prefer eating in own room rather than common dining area
- Action plan:
  - Transfer one aide from day shift to the evening shift
  - Have another aide work 11 AM to 7 PM to help supervise residents
  - Restructure staff dinner hour so that all staff are on unit during residents' dinner hour
  - Increase evening activities in groups
- Follow-up data collected after implementation of action plan:
  - Average of 0.5 falls per day (50% decrease)
  - 30% of falls occur between 4 PM and 8 PM
  - 60% of falls occur in residents' rooms

newer term is utilization management (UM). In the nursing home setting, the UM process usually involves reviewing each resident for Medicare eligibility and certifying residents who meet Medicare criteria for skilled care. The resident's plan of care and outcomes are evaluated periodically by the UR/UM committee, and residents are recertified as appropriate for up to 100 days of skilled care.

The newest trend is to incorporate UM with case management in those facilities where case management exists. Case management is a process to follow high risk, high cost, problem-prone residents throughout their health care episode to ensure consistent, high quality, but cost-effective care. Case managers, therefore, often undertake UM activities as part of their role.

Statistical Analysis

Data collected from the various components of a TQM program must be presented and analyzed by the TQM/CQI committee. The data may be compiled using flow charts, fishbone diagrams, or graphs. A sample graph of data presented in Table 14–1 is shown in Figure 14–2. After analyzing

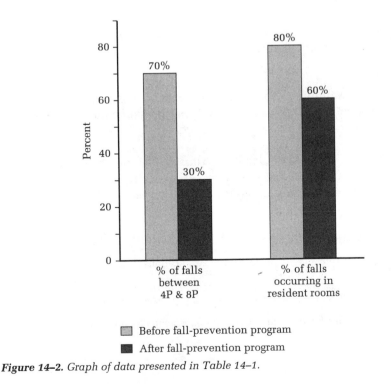

Figure 14–2. Graph of data presented in Table 14–1.

the data and determining that a problem exists or may exist, the committee uses the process previously described under "Risk Management." An action plan is developed, implemented, and re-evaluated for its effectiveness in resolving the identified problem.

Staff Feedback

An important step in CQI that is often overlooked is the need to keep staff at all levels informed of the activities and outcomes of the CQI program. Staff may be asked to collect data but are never told how the data will be used. An action plan may be implemented without any explanation of why the plan is needed. In general, people are more likely to comply and participate in a program if they understand its importance and how it helps improve resident care.

CHAPTER HIGHLIGHTS

Quality assessment is the measurement of quality, usually against predetermined standards.

Quality assurance, considered an outdated term, is a program for monitoring clinical outcomes of residents.

Total quality management is a structured, organization-wide program that serves as an umbrella for its component processes: continuous quality improvement, risk management, performance management, and utilization review (utilization management).

Three different types of standards are those based on structure (focusing on resources needed for care), process (focusing on interventions and care activities), and outcome (focusing on results of care).

REFERENCES AND READINGS

Arikian, V. L. (1991). Total quality management: Applications to nursing service. *Journal of Nursing Administration, 21*(6), 46–59.

Donabedian, A. (1980). *Explorations in quality assessment and monitoring: The definition of quality and approaches to its assessment* (Vol. 1). Ann Arbor, MI: Health Administration Press.

Huber, D. (1996). *Leadership and nursing care management.* Philadelphia: W. B. Saunders.

DISCUSSION QUESTIONS TO PROMOTE CRITICAL THINKING

1. When reviewing infection reports for the residents on your nursing home unit, you note that more and more residents are being placed on antibiotic therapy for urinary tract infections. How might you set up a CQI project to determine if the urinary tract infection rate has really increased?

2. Using the scenario in question #1, what other team members should you involve in this study?

3. Using the scenario in question #1, what data will you need to collect?

15

Legal and Ethical Issues in the Long Term Care Setting

OBJECTIVES

- List four conditions that must be proven for a successful malpractice suit
- Identify key factors that affect ethical decision making
- Describe ethical resources that nurses can use to assist in ethical decision making
- Briefly discuss common ethical dilemmas in long term care

Nurses who work in nursing homes frequently encounter legal and ethical issues related to resident care or employer–employee relationships. These issues vary in scope from relatively minor concerns to very emotional issues, such as "the right to die."

Although legal and ethical issues are related, they are different. A legal issue has a foundation in the law—either local, state, or federal law. Ethics, on the other hand, involves deciding what is right or what an individual ought to do in a given situation. New technology in health care often creates conflicts between ethical decision making and the law. Selected legal and ethical issues are discussed in this chapter.

Legal Aspects Related to Resident Care

Legal issues may arise related to clinical practice or employer–employee relationships. Nursing practice is guided by state law, well-established standards of practice, and the facility's policies and procedures. Employer–employee relationships are guided by a number of federal and state labor laws.

NURSING PRACTICE

Every state has its own nurse practice act that is drafted and passed by the state legislature and signed into law by the governor. This type of law is called *statutory* law. Each state's board of nursing (or similar regulatory body) then develops and circulates regulations that address more specific practice concerns. This type of law is called *regulatory* law. In addition, the board releases interpretive statements and declarative statements that further clarify statutory and regulatory laws.

The nurse licensed and practicing in a given state is obligated to follow these laws or be disciplined by the state's board of nursing. Disciplinary action may include suspending or revoking a nursing license and/or imposing a monetary fine.

A nurse may also be sued for malpractice by a resident, the resident's family, or the resident's guardian. If sued, the plaintiff must prove the following conditions:

1. The nurse had a duty to provide or manage care for the resident.
2. The nurse breached that duty (an error of omission or commission).
3. The resident experienced a negative outcome (harm, injury, and/or suffering).
4. The negative outcome resulted from the nurse's breach of duty (causality).

For example, if a resident falls while under the care of a nurse, the nurse may be sued for malpractice but will not necessarily lose the suit. The key question that is asked is: Did the nurse follow the standard of care? In other words, did the nurse do everything that an ordinary prudent nurse would have done in the same situation? Expert witnesses for the defense of the nurse are in the best position to answer that question and would be used in an arbitration or courtroom hearing.

One of the most valuable tools for defense that any nurse can use is medical record documentation. Most malpractice cases do not get processed for 3 or more years after the event or incident. The nurse may not be able to remember the details of an incident that occurred years ago and will need his or her medical record documentation to assist in the recall of the resident or situation. Documentation is discussed in detail in Chapter 7.

LABOR RELATIONS

Many nurses, whether they are registered nurses or licensed practical/ vocational nurses, are placed in charge of a unit in a nursing home. In this position, part of the nurse's responsibility is supervising other licensed and unlicensed staff members. Charge nurses and nursing administrators must be very familiar with federal and state labor laws, as well as the personnel policies and procedures for the facility or corporation. Regardless of the specific protocols for counseling, disciplining, or terminating an employee, documentation is the most important responsibility of the nurse. Chapter 12 describes employee issues in more detail.

Ethical Decision Making

All health professionals use an ethical decision-making process, also known as ethical reasoning, when faced with an ethical dilemma in clinical practice.

FACTORS AFFECTING ETHICAL DECISION MAKING

Many factors can affect how a nurse makes an ethical decision in long term care. These factors can be divided into three categories, according to which they are associated with the nurse, the environment, or the task (Bosek & Savage, 1995).

Nurse factors are those belonging to the person of the nurse, such as gender, age, self-concept, values, and beliefs. For example, for the nurse who believes that elderly people should receive aggressive treatment measures regardless of their age or overall health, issues such as withholding tube feedings and do not resuscitate orders create major ethical dilemmas.

Environmental factors may be related to the facility or related to the community. Facility-related factors that influence decision making might include facility philosophy, policies and procedures, time limitations, and available technology or equipment. For example, a resident may be more comfortable staying in a nursing home even though the technology that could prolong the resident's life is not available in that setting. An example of a community factor is public sentiment about how health care resources should be allocated.

Task factors are those less tangible factors that nurses use to help in the decision-making process. Sometimes nurses use "rules" they learned in nursing school, such as "Don't give opioids to elderly people because they might cause respiratory depression." As a result of learning this rule, nurses often undermedicate elderly residents who are experiencing acute or chronic pain. Other factors that can enter into the ethical decision-making process are the perceived costs and benefits associated with a possible intervention.

DECISION-MAKING PROCESS

The steps for ethical decision making are similar to the steps of the nursing process. For each decision, the nurse:

1. Identifies the ethical problem
2. Lists alternative actions
3. Identifies probable outcomes for each alternative action
4. Implements one of the alternatives
5. Evaluates the outcome of the action taken

While this process may seem fairly easy, it is often difficult to use this process in an actual clinical situation. The factors described in the previous section make the process more complex, especially the nurse's values and beliefs.

ETHICAL RESOURCES

A number of resources are available to help nurses and the rest of the health care team make decisions regarding ethical dilemmas. Examples are the ANA Code for Nurses, the institution's patient care advisory committee, medical and related literature, and people resources.

American Nurses' Association Code for Nurses

The Code for Nurses, developed by the American Nurses' Association (1985), is a code of ethics that is currently being revised. The code is actually a list of tenets or principles to guide nurses in their ethical decision making.

Patient Care Advisory Committee

The patient care advisory committee (PCAC) is an interdisciplinary group of people who have the responsibility of advising health professionals, when necessary, regarding ethical decisions. Committee membership typically includes nurses, physicians, administrators, social workers, clergy, attorneys, and lay persons. By federal law, all nursing homes must have a PCAC to determine ethical policies and provide advice when asked.

Literature and People Resources

As they struggle with ethical situations, several other resources are available to assist nurses in long term care facilities. During the past 10 years, many articles in professional journals and books have been written to help nurses with ethical dilemmas. Supervisors and administrators can also provide assistance when the nurse is challenged with an ethical situation.

The state or local ombudsman (through the office on aging) can also provide support or advice to a facility. The ombudsman's role is to ensure protection of residents' rights. In large corporations or facilities, an ethics consultant may be available for advice in difficult situations.

COMMON ETHICAL ISSUES

The nurse employed in long term care faces numerous ethical situations or issues. Some of the most common dilemmas include advance directives, do not resuscitate orders, competence, tube feedings, confidentiality, and unethical professional conduct.

Advance Directives

Advance directives provide a way for people to indicate their decisions about future medical care. A written advance directive is a legal document that specifies what the individual would prefer regarding life and health decisions in the event that the individual cannot express his or her wishes. The Patient Self Determination Act of 1990 requires that all residents admitted to a nursing home or hospital be informed about the availability of advance directives. If the resident already has a written advance directive, a copy is placed in the medical record and in the administrative file for reference when needed.

Most states allow two common types of directives: the living will and the durable power of attorney for health care. The *living will*, sometimes referred to as the "death with dignity will," allows people to specify their wishes regarding life-sustaining medical care in case they are imminently dying of a terminal illness or condition. Most states require that "imminent death" be consistent with the hospice definition, which usually means that the expected life span is 3 to 6 months; however, each state's definition differs. The nurse must be aware of the laws in his or her state.

The *durable power of attorney for health care* (DPOA), also called the durable medical power of attorney, allows people to identify someone to make health and life decisions for them if they are unable to express their own decisions; list medical treatments they would never want performed; and specify treatment should they be in a coma or persistent vegetative state. Each state's DPOA varies somewhat, and the nurse must be familiar with the legal document that is recognized in the state where she or he works. A sample DPOA is found in Figure 15–1.

In recent years, *verbal* directives have started to be recognized as legitimate types of advance directives. If the resident has no written direc-

DURABLE POWER OF ATTORNEY FOR HEALTH CARE

Power of Attorney made this _____ day of _____, 19____

    1. I, the undersigned hereby appoint (insert name and address of agent)

_____

as agent to act for me and in my name to make any and all decisions for me concerning my personal care, medical treatment, hospitalization and health care and to require, withhold or withdraw any type of medical treatment or procedure, even though my death may ensue. My agent shall have the same access to my medical records that I have, including the right to disclose the contents to others. My agent shall also have full power to make a disposition of any part or all of my body for medical purposes, authorize an autopsy and direct the disposition of my remains. (Neither the attending physician nor any other health care provider may act as your agent.)

    2. The powers granted above shall be subject to the following rules or limitations (if none, leave blank):

_____

_____

(The subject of life-sustaining treatment is of particular importance. For your convenience in dealing with that subject some general statements concerning the withholding or removal of life-sustaining treatment are set forth below. If you agree with one of these statements, you may initial that statement; but do not initial more than one.)

          (I do not want my life to be prolonged nor do I want life-sustaining treatment
          (to be provided or continued if my agent believes the burdens of the treatment
          (outweigh the expected benefits. I want my agent to consider the relief of
          (suffering the expense involved and the quality as well as the possible extension
_____(of my life in making decisions concerning life-sustaining treatment.

          (I want my life to be prolonged and I want life-sustaining treatment to be
          (provided or continued unless I am in a coma which my attending physician
          (believes to be irreversible, in accordance with reasonable medical standards at
          (the time of reference. If and when I have suffered irreversible coma, I want
_____(life-sustaining treatment to be withheld or discontinued.

          (I want my life to be prolonged to the greatest extent possible without regard to
_____(my condition, the chances I have for recovery or the cost of the procedures.

    3. This power of attorney shall become effective on _____

Figure 15–1. An example of a durable power of attorney for health care.

tive but has told family members or friends of his or her wishes for health care, the facility can honor those directives in many states. Some states also have a next-of-kin law that specifies in which order the physician can obtain consent for certain procedures or treatments when these are not specified in advance by the resident. While not usually required, health professionals typically obtain next-of-kin consent to minimize the risk of malpractice suits.

Do Not Resuscitate Orders

Cardiopulmonary resuscitation (CPR) was developed to treat witnessed cardiac arrests in otherwise healthy young people. However, the use of CPR has expanded. In cases of individuals with terminal illnesses or advanced age, the use of CPR has been questioned. The quality of life issue has entered the debate about who should be resuscitated and under what conditions.

The nurse and physician should discuss do not resuscitate (DNR) orders with the residents or their legal guardians in a nursing home setting. The presence of a written advance directive does *not* automatically indicate a DNR order. Each long term care facility should have policies regarding DNR orders and how they are to be interpreted.

Competence

When issues of competence are raised, two types of competence must be considered—legal and clinical competence. *Legal* competence is governed by each state. In most states, a person is legally competent if he or she is 18 years of age or older (unless a pregnant or married minor) and has not been declared incompetent by a court of law.

If an individual has been declared *incompetent*, the court appoints a legal guardian to make decisions for the individual. A guardian of person can make decisions related to health and life. A guardian of property can make financial decisions.

Clinical competence refers to a person's ability to make sound decisions with rationales. The nurse or other health professional must assess the individual for the ability to identify a problem or issue, weigh the risks and benefits of the possible solutions, and select a solution that best meets his or her needs. If a resident is not clinically competent, next of kin or the resident's legal representative may be consulted.

Tube Feeding

Total enteral nutrition, often referred to as a tube feeding, has been another source of debate in health care. A number of ethical questions have been raised with respect to this procedure: Does the benefit of long term tube feeding outweigh its risks? Do comfort measures include nutrition? Is tube feeding an extraordinary treatment measure that should not be performed in the case of terminal illness and imminent death? Is malnutrition painful?

While no one seems to have the definitive answers to these questions, it is not uncommon for individuals to state that they do *not* want to have life sustained by tube feeding if they are terminally ill, in a coma, or in a persistent vegetative state. The American Academy of Neurology considers tube feedings for nutrition and hydration as therapy that residents or surrogate decision makers may refuse (Bernat, Goldstein, & Viste, 1996).

Other issues that arise related to total enteral nutrition include respect for life, quality of life, and allocation of resources. Nurses who work in the nursing home setting must examine their feelings about tube feedings and discuss them with the health care team.

Confidentiality

In nursing school, every student learns that confidentiality, privacy, and dignity are essential for the individuals they care for. These characteristics are also part of the ANA Code for Nurses, described earlier. However, in clinical practice it is often very easy to forget their importance.

In the nursing home setting, nursing staff become so familiar with the residents in their homelike setting that they may unintentionally discuss information about a resident using his or her name in a public place, such as the elevator or employee lounge. The nurse should set an example to the rest of the staff by being a role model and reminding them of the need for resident confidentiality.

Resident privacy and dignity may also be unintentionally sacrificed. Doors to residents' rooms and curtains must be closed during a bath or other procedure. The staff should also respect the resident by knocking on his or her door before entering. The fact that a long term care facility is a home for residents needs to be appreciated and respected. Discussing a competent resident's condition with family or significant others without the resident's permission is also an invasion of privacy.

Unethical Professional Conduct

Although it is not a common occurrence, the nurse may encounter another nurse, staff member, or health care professional whose conduct does not meet the standard of practice. The third tenet of the ANA Code of Ethics addresses the responsibility of the nurse to protect clients (residents) from health care professionals who engage in illegal, unethical, or incompetent practice.

For example, if a nurse sees a staff member physically or mentally abusing a resident, he or she is obligated to protect the resident and report the staff member following the appropriate chain of command in the organization. The incident must be documented and disciplinary action taken against the abusive staff member by the facility. The nursing home must contact the local police to investigate the incident.

CHAPTER HIGHLIGHTS

Four conditions must be met in a malpractice suit: a duty; a breach of duty; harm, injury, or suffering (negative outcome); and a cause-and-effect relationship between the breach and the negative outcome.

Many factors affect a nurse's ethical decision-making process, including those relating to the nurse, the environment, and the task.

Resources available to the nurse to assist in ethical decision making include the ANA Code of Ethics, the patient care advisory committee, professional health literature, the ombudsman, and ethics consultants.

Common ethical dilemmas that nurses in long term care encounter include issues related to advance directives, do not resuscitate orders, competence, tube feeding, and confidentiality. Less commonly, the nurse may observe unethical professional conduct.

REFERENCES AND READINGS

American Nurses Association. (1985). *ANA code for nurses.* Washington, DC: Author.
Bernat, J. L., Goldstein, M. L., & Viste, K. M. (1996). The neurologist and the dying patient. *Neurology, 46,* 598–599.
Bosek, M., & Savage, T. (1995). Ethics. In D. Ignatavicius, L. Workman, & M. Mishler (Eds.), *Medical-surgical nursing: A nursing process approach* (pp. 81–100). Philadelphia: W. B. Saunders.

DISCUSSION QUESTIONS TO PROMOTE CRITICAL THINKING

1. Although not diagnosed with dementia, an elderly resident is sometimes confused, particularly in the evening. He has not been declared legally incompetent. Every warm-weather afternoon the resident takes a walk outside the facility and crosses a busy highway to shop at a local convenience store. When consulted, the ombudsman states that it is the resident's right to go where he wants to go as long as he is physically able. Is there a way to resolve this ethical dilemma?

2. In this scenario, what documentation would you need to protect your practice from a legal perspective?

3. If the resident is injured during his walk to the store, could you and your facility be successfully sued for malpractice? Why or why not?

APPENDIX **A**

Common Laboratory Tests and Their Clinical Significance

SERUM LABORATORY TEST	NORMAL ADULT RANGE	CLINICAL SIGNIFICANCE

Acid phosphatase	0.11–0.60 U/L	*Decreased:*
		  No significance
		Increased:
		  Prostate cancer
		  Multiple myeloma

Alanine amino-
  transferase (ALT)
	5–35 IU/L
	Elderly: may be
	  slightly increased
		Decreased:
		  No significance
		Increased:
		  Hepatitis
		  Cirrhosis
		  Hepatic necrosis
		  Hepatotoxic drugs
		  Hepatic tumor

Alkaline
  phosphatase
	30–85 ImU/mL
	Elderly: may be
	  slightly increased
		Decreased:
		  Hypothyroidism
		  Malnutrition
		  Hypophosphatemia
		Increased:
		  Cirrhosis
		  Paget's disease
		  Liver disease
		  Metastatic bone disease
		  Healing fractures
		  Hyperparathyroidism

Ammonia	15–110 µg/dL or
	47–65 mmol/L
		Decreased:
		  No significance
		Increased:
		  Primary hepatic disease
		  Hepatic coma

(table continues)

SERUM LABORATORY TEST	NORMAL ADULT RANGE	CLINICAL SIGNIFICANCE
		Severe heart disease with congestive hepatomegaly
Amylase	56–190 IU/L, 80–150 Somogyi units/L, or 25–125 U/L	*Decreased:* No significance *Increased:* Acute pancreatitis Perforated bowel or stomach Chronic relapsing pancreatitis
Antinuclear antibody (ANA)	<1:8	*Decreased:* No significance *Increased:* Systemic lupus erythematosus Rheumatoid arthritis Chronic hepatitis Progressive systemic sclerosis Polymyositis Dermatomyositis Sjögren's syndrome Leukemia Myasthenia gravis
Arterial blood gases (ABGs)	pH: 7.34–7.45	*Decreased:* Acidosis (metabolic or respiratory) *Increased:* Alkalosis (metabolic or respiratory)
	PO_2: 90–100 mm Hg **Elderly:** as low as 80 mm Hg	*Decreased:* Chronic or acute respiratory disease Cardiac disease Pulmonary embolus Fat embolism syndrome (FES) *Increased:* Not significant, most likely the result of oxygen administration
	PCO_2: 32–45 mm Hg **Elderly:** may be slightly increased	*Decreased:* Alkalosis (usually respiratory) *Increased:* Acidosis (usually respiratory)
	HCO_3: 20–26 mEq/L	*Decreased:* Metabolic acidosis *Increased:* Renal compensation of respiratory acidosis
Aspartate amino-transferase (AST)	8–20 U/L or 5–40 IU/L	*Decreased:* Diabetic ketoacidosis

SERUM LABORATORY TEST	NORMAL ADULT RANGE	CLINICAL SIGNIFICANCE

		Increased:
		   Myocardial infarction
		   Hepatitis
		   Cirrhosis
		   Acute pancreatitis
		   Multiple trauma
		   Primary muscle diseases
		   Hepatic necrosis

Bilirubin	Total: 0.1–1.0 mg/dL
	   or 5.1–17.0 mmol/L
	 Indirect: 0.2–0.8 mg/dL
	   or 3.4–12.0 mmol/L
	
	 Direct: 0.1–0.3 mg/dL
	   or 1.7–5.1 mmol/L
		Decreased:
		   No significance
		 Increased:
		   Cirrhosis
		   Hepatitis
		   Hemolytic jaundice
		   Bile duct obstruction

Blood urea nitrogen	10–20 mg/dL or
	 3.6–7.1 mmol/L
	
	 Elderly: Increased
	 (may be as high as
	 69 mg/dL)
		Decreased:
		   Overhydration
		   Malnutrition
		 Increased:
		   Dehydration
		   Renal disease
		   Excessive dietary protein
		   Liver failure
		   Catabolic state

CA-125 tumor marker	0–35 U/mL	*Decreased:*
		   No significance
		 Increased:
		   Ovarian cancer
		   Colon cancer
		   Upper GI cancers
		   Cirrhosis
		   Peritonitis
		   Metastatic peritoneal cancer
		   Endometriosis

CA 15-3 tumor marker	< 22 U/mL	*Decreased:*
		   No significance
		 Increased:
		   Metastatic breast cancer

CA 19-9 tumor marker	< 37 U/mL	*Decreased:*
		   No significance
		 Increased:
		   Pancreatic cancer
		   Hepatobiliary cancer
		   Gastric cancer
		   Colon cancer
		   Pancreatitis
		   Cholelithiasis

Calcium	4.5–5.5 mEq/L
	   or 8.0–10.5 mg/dL
	 Elderly: Slightly
	 decreased
		Decreased:
		   Osteoporosis
		   Malabsorption
		   Renal failure
		   Acute pancreatitis
		   Hyperphosphatemia

(table continues)

SERUM LABORATORY TEST	NORMAL ADULT RANGE	CLINICAL SIGNIFICANCE
		Removal or dysfunction of parathyroid glands Vitamin D toxicity *Increased:* Renal failure (oliguric phase) Hyperparathyroidism Hypophosphatemia Malignancy Vitamin D deficiency
Carcinoembryonic antigen (CEA)	< 5 ng/mL or 0–2.5 µg/L	*Decreased:* No significance *Increased:* Cancer (GI, breast, lung) Inflammation (colitis, cholecystitis, pancreatitis) Cirrhosis Peptic ulcer
Cholesterol	150–200 mg/dL or 3.9–6.5 mmol/L	*Decreased:* Malnutrition Malabsorption Liver disease *Increased:* Hyperlipidemia Uncontrolled diabetes mellitus High-cholesterol diet Atherosclerosis
Creatinine	0.5–1.2 mg/dL or 44–97 mol/L **Elderly:** slightly increased	*Decreased:* No significance
Creatinine kinase (CK)	Total: 10–70 U/mL CK-MM: 100% CK-MB: 0% CK-BB: 0%	*Decreased:* No significance *Increased:* Acute myocardial infarction (total and CK-MB) Muscular dystrophy (total and CK-MM) Pulmonary infarction (total and CK-BB) Polymyositis Dermatomyositis
Glucose (fasting blood sugar [FBS])	70–105 mg/dL or 3.9–5.8 mmol/L **Elderly:** increased range after 50 yr	*Decreased:* Hypoglycemia Excessive insulin *Increased:* Hyperglycemia Excessive IV infusion of glucose or dextrose solutions Prolonged corticosteroid use Pancreatic disease

SERUM LABORATORY TEST	NORMAL ADULT RANGE	CLINICAL SIGNIFICANCE

Hematocrit	Females: 37%–47%
	Males: 42%–52%
	Elderly: may be
	  slightly decreased
		Decreased:
		  Blood loss
		  Anemia
		  Renal failure
		  Immunocompromised state
		  Overhydration
		Increased:
		  Dehydration
		  Polycythemia vera

Hemoglobin	Females: 12–16 g/dL
	  or 7.4–9.9 mmol/L
	Males: 14–18 g/L or
	  8.7–11.2 mmol/L
	Elderly: slightly
	  decreased
		Decreased:
		  Blood loss
		  Anemia
		  Renal failure
		  Immunocompromised
		    state
		Increased:
		  Polycythemia vera
		  Chronic pulmonary
		    disease

Iron level & total
  iron binding
  capacity (TIBC)
	Iron: 60–190 µg/L
	  or 13–31 mmol/L
	TIBC: 25–420 µg/L
	  or 45–73 mmol/L
		Decreased:
		  Iron-deficiency anemia
		  Chronic blood loss
		  Neoplasia
		  Iron-deficient diet
		  Malabsorption
		  Hypoproteinemia (TIBC)
		Increased:
		  Hemolytic anemias
		  Hepatic necrosis
		  Polycythemia vera

Lactate dehydro-
  genase (LDH)
	45–90 U/L,
	  115–225 IU/L,
	  or 0.4–1.7 mmol/L
	LDH-1: 17–27%
	LDH-2: 27–37%
	LDH-3: 18–25%
	LDH-4: 3–8%
	LDH-5: 0–5%
		Decreased:
		  No significance
		Increased:
		  Myocardial
		    infarction
		  Pulmonary diseases
		    (e.g., infarction)
		  Skeletal muscle disease
		    and trauma
		  Muscular dystrophy
		  Hepatitis
		  Hemolytic anemias
		  Intestinal infarction
		  Pancreatitis

Lipase	0–110 units/L
	  or 0–417 U/L
		Decreased:
		  No significance
		Increased:
		  Acute pancreatitis
		  Chronic relapsing
		    pancreatitis
		  Acute cholecystitis

(*table continues*)

SERUM LABORATORY TEST	NORMAL ADULT RANGE	CLINICAL SIGNIFICANCE

Partial thromboplastin time (PTT); activated thrombo-plastin time (aPTT)	PTT: 60–70 sec
	
	aPPT: 30– 40 sec
		Decreased:
		  Clotting disorder
		  Extensive cancer
		Increased:
		  Bleeding disorder
		  Anticoagulant therapy
		    (heparin)
		  Liver disease

Platelet count (thrombocyte count)	150,000–400,000/mm^3
	  or 150–400 × 10^7/L
		Decreased:
		  Platelet destruction
		  Hemmorhage
		  Thrombocytopenia purpura
		  Leukemias
		  Liver disease
		  Bone marrow suppression
		  Disseminated intravascular
		    dissemination (DIC)
		  Systemic lupus
		    erythematosus
		  Hemolytic anemias
		Increased:
		  Malignant disorders
		  Polycythemia vera
		  Postsplenectomy syndromes

Prostate-specific antigen (PSA)	< 4 ng/mL	*Decreased:*
		  No significance
		Increased:
		  Prostate cancer
		  Prostatitis
		  Benign prostatic
		    hypertrophy

Protein	Total: 6–8 g/dL
	Albumin: 3.2–4.5
	  g/dL
	Globulin: 2.3–3.4
	  g/dL
		Decreased:
		  Malnutrition
		  Liver disease
		  Malabsorption
		  Third space losses (e.g.,
		    ascites)
		Increased:
		  Hemoconcentration

Prothrombin time (Protime, PT)	11–12.5 sec, 85%–
	100%
		Decreased:
		  Clotting disorder
		  Extensive cancer
		Increased:
		  Bleeding disorder
		  Anticoagulant therapy
		    (warfarin)

Potassium	3.5–5.0 mEq/L or
	3.5–5.0 mmol/L
		Decreased:
		  Prolonged diuretic or
		    corticosteroid use
		  Cushing's syndrome
		  Metabolic alkalosis
		  Loss of gastrointestinal
		    fluids

SERUM LABORATORY TEST	NORMAL ADULT RANGE	CLINICAL SIGNIFICANCE
		Increased: Excessive potassium intake Addison's disease Hemolysis Extensive tissue damage
Red blood cell (RBC) count	Male: 4.7–6.1 million/mm^3 Female: 4.2–5.4 million/mm^3	*Decreased:* Hemorrhage Hemolysis Anemias Leukemias Chronic illness Bone marrow suppression Renal failure Multiple myeloma Overhydration Dietary deficiencies Connective tissue diseases *Increased:* Polycythemia vera Dehydration/hemo-concentration High altitude
Sodium	136–145 mEq/L or 136–145 mmol/L	*Decreased:* Diuretic therapy Excessive diaphoresis Renal disease (polyuric phase) Loss of gastric fluids *Increased:* Hyperaldosteronism Renal failure (oliguric phase) Cushing's syndrome Prolonged corticosteroid therapy
Thyroid-stimulating hormone (TSH)	2–10 mU/ml	*Decreased:* Pituitary dysfunction Hyperthyroidism *Increased:* Primary hypothyroidism Thyroiditis
Thyroxine (T4)	4–11 µg/dL	*Decreased:* Hypothyroidism Protein malnutrition *Increased:* Hyperthyroidism Acute thyroiditis
Triglycerides	35–160 mg/dL or 0.35–1.6 g/L	*Decreased:* Malabsorption Malnutrition *Increased:* Hyperlipidemia

(*table continues*)

SERUM LABORATORY TEST	NORMAL ADULT RANGE	CLINICAL SIGNIFICANCE
		Poorly controlled diabetes mellitus Atherosclerosis High-fat, high-carbohydrate diet
Uric acid	2.0–8.5 mg/dL or 0.09–0.48 mmol/L **Elderly:** may be slightly increased	*Decreased:* Wilson's disease *Increased:* Gout Multiple myeloma Metastatic cancer Renal failure Alcoholism Leukemias
White blood cell (WBC) count	5000–10,000 cells/mm^3	*Decreased:* Immune disorders, such as acquired immuno-deficiency syndrome Immunocompromised state Chemotherapy *Increased:* Infection Leukemias

Reprinted with permission from Ignatavicius, DD, and Hausman, KA: Pocket Companion for Medical-Surgical Nursing, 2nd ed. Philadelphia, W.B. Saunders, 1995.

APPENDIX B

Preadmission Screening/Annual Resident Review (PASARR) Form

DEPARTMENT OF HEALTH AND
MENTAL HYGIENE
PREADMISSION SCREENING AND ANNUAL
RESIDENT REVIEW (PASARR)
LEVEL I ID SCREEN FOR
MENTAL ILLNESS AND MENTAL RETARDATION
OR RELATED CONDITIONS

Check one ___PAS

___ARR

NOTE: This form must be completed for all applicants to nursing facilities (NF) which participate in the Maryland Medical Assistance Program, regardless of applicant's payment source.

Last Name:_____ First Name:_____ MI:___

Date of Birth:_____SSN:_____ Sex: Male____Female_____

Actual/Requested Nursing Facility Adm. Date:_____

Current Location of Individual:_____

Address:_____ City/State_____ Zip:_____

Contact Person:_____ Title/Relationship_____

Telephone No._____

A. EXEMPTED HOSPITAL DISCHARGE

1. Is the individual admitted to a NF
directly from a hospital after receiving
acute inpatient care?   Yes ☐   No ☐

2. Does the individual require NF services
for the condition for which he received
care in the hospital?   Yes ☐   No ☐

3. Has the attending physician certified
before admission to the NF that the
resident is likely to require less than
30 days NF services?   Yes ☐   No ☐

IF ALL THREE QUESTIONS ARE ANSWERED YES, FURTHER
    SCREENING IS *NOT* REQUIRED (PLEASE SIGN AND DATE BELOW)
IF ANY QUESTION IS ANSWERED NO, THE REMAINDER OF THE
    FORM MUST BE COMPLETED AS DIRECTED.

IF THE STAY EXTENDS FOR 30 DAYS OR MORE, A NEW SCREEN
    AND ARR MUST BE PERFORMED WITHIN 40 DAYS OF
    ADMISSION.

Signature_____ Title_____ Date_____

B. MENTAL RETARDATION (MR) AND RELATED CONDITIONS
    (see definitions)

1. Does the individual have a diagnosis of
MR or related condition? If yes, specify
diagnosis_____   Yes ☐   No ☐

2. Is there any history of MR or related
condition in the individual's past,
prior to age 22?   Yes ☐   No ☐

3. Is there any presenting evidence
   (cognitive or behavior functions) that
   may indicate that the individual has MR
   or related conditions?   Yes ☐   No ☐

4. Is the individual being referred by, and
   deemed eligible for services by an
   agency which serves persons with MR
   or related conditions?   Yes ☐   No ☐

Is the individual considered to have MR
or a Related Condition? If the answer is
Yes to one or more of the above, check
"Yes." If the answers are *No* to all of the
above check "No."   Yes ☐   No ☐

_____

4345-1 Rev. 4/93

Name_____

C. SERIOUS MENTAL ILLNESS (MI) (see definitions)

1. Diagnosis. Does the individual have a
   major mental disorder? If yes, list
   diagnosis and DSM III-R
   Code_____   Yes ☐   No ☐

2. Level of Impairment. Has the disorder
   resulted in serious functional limitations
   in major life activities within the past
   3–6 months (e.g., interpersonal
   functioning, concentration, persistence
   and pace; or adaptation to change)?   Yes ☐   No ☐

3. Recent treatment. In the past 2 years,
   has individual had more than one
   inpatient psychiatric admission or an
   episode of significant disruption to the
   normal living situation where supportive

services were required to maintain
functioning at home or in a residential
treatment environment or which resulted
in intervention by housing or law
enforcement officials?   Yes ☐   No ☐

- -

Is the individual considered to have a
SERIOUS MENTAL ILLNESS? If the answer is
Yes to all 3 of the above, check "Yes." If the
response is *No* to one or more of the above,
check "No."   Yes ☐   No ☐

If the individual *is* considered to have MI or MR or a related condition,
complete Part D of this form. Otherwise, skip Part D and sign below.

D. CATEGORICAL ADVANCE GROUP DETERMINATIONS

1. Is the individual being admitted for
   convalescent care not to exceed 120 days
   due to an acute physical illness which
   required hospitalization and does not
   meet all criteria for an exempt hospital
   discharge (described in Part A)?   Yes ☐   No ☐

2. Does the individual have a terminal
   illness (life expectancy of less than
   six months) as certified by a physician?   Yes ☐   No ☐

3. Does the individual have a severe
   physical illness which results in a level
   of impairment so severe that the
   individual could not be expected to
   benefit from specialized services?   Yes ☐   No ☐

4. Is this individual being provisionally
   admitted pending further assessment
   due to an emergency situation requiring
   protective services? The stay will not
   exceed 7 days.   Yes ☐   No ☐

5. Is the individual being admitted for a
   stay not to exceed 14 days to provide
   respite?   Yes ☐   No ☐

If any answer to Part D is "Yes," complete the Categorical Advance Group Determination Evaluation Report and attach. Additionally, if questions 1, 2 or 3 are checked "Yes," or if *all* answers in Part D are "No," the individual must be referred to GES for a Level II evaluation.

I certify that the above information is correct to the best of my knowledge. If the initial ID screen is positive and a GES Level II evaluation is required, a copy of the ID screen has been provided to the applicant/resident and legal representative.

Name & Title_____ Date_____

FOR POSITIVE ID SCREENS, NOT COVERED UNDER CATEGORICAL DETERMINATIONS, Check below.

_____ This applicant has been cleared by the Department for nursing facility admission.

_____ This resident has been reviewed as part of the annual resident review process.

Local GES Office_____ Contact_____ Date_____

DHMH-4345-2 Rev. 4/93

Minimum Data Set (MDS) and Resident Assessment Protocol (RAP) Summary

07/31/1996   51-1166
                    Numeric Identifier ——————————

MINIMUM DATA SET (MDS) - VERSION 2.0
FOR NURSING HOME RESIDENT ASSESSMENT AND CARE SCREENING
BASIC ASSESSMENT TRACKING FORM

SECTION AA. IDENTIFICATION INFORMATION	GENERAL INSTRUCTIONS

GENERAL INSTRUCTIONS
Complete this information for submission with all full and quarterly assessments (Admission, Annual, Significant Change, State or Medicare required assessments, or Quarterly Reviews, etc.).

1. RESIDENT NAME ⊙
a. (First)   b. (Middle initial)   c. (Last)   d. (Jr./Sr.)

2. GENDER ⊙
1. Male   2. Female | 2 |

3. BIRTHDATE ⊙
| 0 | 3 | — | 2 | 8 | — | 1 | 9 | 0 | 2 |
Month   Day   Year

4. RACE/ETHNICITY ⊙
1. American Indian/Alaskan Native   4. Hispanic
2. Asian/Pacific Islander   5. White, not of Hispanic origin
3. Black, not of Hispanic origin | 5 |

5. SOCIAL SECURITY AND MEDICARE NUMBERS (C in 1st box if non Med. no.) ⊙
a. Social Security Number
| 2 | 1 | 8 | — | 5 | 6 | — | 8 | 9 | 8 | 7 |
b. Medicare number (or comparable railroad insurance number)
| 1 | 7 | 9 | 0 | 9 | 0 | 1 | 1 | 0 | D | 2 |

6. FACILITY PROVIDER NO. ⊙
a. State No.
| 2 | 1 | 5 | 1 | 5 | 1 | | | | | |
b. Federal No.
| | | 5 | 2 | 1 | 3 | 3 | 9 | 4 | 5 | 8 | | |

7. MEDICAID NO. (" + " if pending, "N" if not a Medicaid recipient) ⊙

8. REASONS FOR ASSESSMENT [Note - Other codes do not apply to this form]
a. Primary reason for assessment
1. Admission assessment (required by day 14)
2. Annual assessment
3. Significant change in status assessment
4. Significant correction of prior assessment
5. Quarterly review assessment
0. *NONE ABOVE* | 1 |
b. *Special codes for use with supplemental assessment types in Case Mix demonstration states or other states where required*
1. 5 day assessment
2. 30 day assessment
3. 60 day assessment
4. Quarterly assessment using full MDS form
5. Readmission / return assessment
6. Other state required assessment

9. SIGNATURES OF PERSONS COMPLETING THESE ITEMS:
7/11/96
a. Signatures   Title   Date
b.   Date

⊙ = Key items for computerized resident tracking
▢ = When box blank, must enter number or letter
a. = When letter in box, check if condition applies
Code "-" if information unavailable or unknown

TRIGGER LEGEND

1	- Delirium	10A	- Activities (Revise)
2	- Cognitive Loss/Dementia	10B	- Activities (Review)
3	- Visual Function	11	- Falls
4	- Communication	12	- Nutritional Status
5A	- ADL-Rehabilitation	13	- Feeding Tubes
5B	- ADL-Maintenance	14	- Dehydration / Fluid Maintenance
6	- Urinary Incontinence and Indwelling Catheter	15	- Dental Care
7	- Psychosocial Well-Being	16	- Pressure Ulcers
8	- Mood State	17	- Psychotropic Drug Use
9	- Behavioral Symptoms	18	- Physical Restraints

Resident _____ 07/31/1996 _____ Numeric Identifier _____ 51-1166 _____

MINIMUM DATA SET (MDS) - VERSION 2.0
FOR NURSING HOME RESIDENT ASSESSMENT AND CARE SCREENING
BACKGROUND (FACE SHEET) INFORMATION AT ADMISSION

SECTION AB. DEMOGRAPHIC INFORMATION

1.	DATE OF ENTRY	Date the stay began. Note - Does not include readmission if record was closed at time of temporary discharge to hospital, etc. In such cases, use prior admission date.

0	7	—	1	7	—	1	9	9	6
Month			Day			Year			

2.	ADMITTED FROM (AT ENTRY)	1. Private home/apt. with no home health services 2. Private home/apt. with home health services 3. Board and care/assisted living/group home 4. Nursing home 5. Acute care hospital 6. Psychiatric hospital, MR/DD facility 7. Rehabilitation hospital 8. Other	4
3.	LIVED ALONE (PRIOR TO ENTRY)	0. No 1. Yes 2. In other facility	0
4.	ZIP CODE OF PRIOR PRIMARY RESIDENCE	2 0 7 3 5	
5.	RESIDEN-TIAL HISTORY 5 YEARS PRIOR TO ENTRY	(Check all settings resident lived in during 5 years prior to date of entry given in item AB1 above.)	
		Prior stay at this nursing home	a.
		Stay in other nursing home	b. x
		Other residential facility - board and care home, assisted living, group home	c.
		MH/psychiatric setting	d.
		MR/DD setting	e.
		NONE OF ABOVE	f.
	LIFETIME OCCUPA-TION(S) (Put "/" between two occupations)	HOUSEWIFE	
7.	EDUCATION (Highest level completed)	1. No schooling 5. Technical or trade school 2. 8th grade/less 6. Some college 3. 9 -11 grades 7. Bachelor's degree 4. High school 8. Graduate degree	7
8.	LANGUAGE	(Code for correct response) a. Primary Language 0. English 1. Spanish 2. French 3. Other	0
		b. If other, specify	
9.	MENTAL HEALTH HISTORY	Does resident's RECORD indicate any history of mental retardation, mental illness, or developmental disability problem? 0. No 1. Yes	0
10.	CONDITIONS RELATED TO MR/DD STATUS	(Check all conditions that are related to MR/DD status that were manifested before age 22, and are likely to continue indefinitely)	
		Not applicable - no MR/DD (Skip to AB11)	a. x
		MR/DD with organic condition	b.
		Down's syndrome	c.
		Autism	d.
		Epilepsy	e.
		Other organic condition related to MR/DD	
		MR/DD with no organic condition	f.
11.	DATE BACK-GROUND INFORMA-TION COMPLETED		

0	7	—	1	7	—	1	9	9	6
Month			Day			Year			

SECTION AC. CUSTOMARY ROUTINE

1.	CUSTOMARY ROUTINE	(Check all that apply. If all information UNKNOWN, check last box only.)

(In year prior to DATE OF ENTRY to this nursing, home, or year last in community if now being admitted from another nursing home)

CYCLE OF DAILY EVENTS	
Stays up late at night (e.g., after 9 pm)	a.
Naps regularly during day (at least 1 hour)	b. x
Goes out 1 + days a week	c.
Stays busy with hobbies, reading, or fixed daily routine	d. x
Spends most of time alone or watching TV	e.
Moves independently indoors (with appliances, if used)	f. x
Use of tobacco products at least daily	g.
NONE OF ABOVE	h.
EATING PATTERNS	
Distinct food preferences	i. x
Eats between meals all or most days	j. x
Use of alcoholic beverage(s) at least weekly	k.
NONE OF ABOVE	l.
ADL PATTERNS	
In bedclothes much of day	m.
Wakens to toilet all or most nights	n.
Has irregular bowel movement pattern	o.
Showers for bathing	p. x
Bathing in PM	q.
NONE OF ABOVE	r.
INVOLVEMENT PATTERNS	
Daily contact with relatives/close friends	s.
Usually attends church, temple, synagogue (etc.)	t.
Finds strength in faith	u.
Daily animal companion/presence	v.
Involved in group activities	w. x
NONE OF ABOVE	x. x
UNKNOWN - Resident / family unable to provide information	y.

END

SECTION AD. FACE SHEET SIGNATURES

SIGNATURES OF PERSONS COMPLETING FACE SHEET: 1/17/96

a. Signature of RN Assessment Coordinator			Date
b. Signatures	Title	Sections	Date
c.			Date
d.			Date
e.			Date
f.			Date
g.			Date

☐ = When box blank, must enter number or letter

[a.] = When letter in box, check if condition applies

ode "-" if information unavailable or unknown

NOTE: Normally, the MDS Face Sheet is completed once, when an individual first enters the facility. However, the face sheet is also required if the person is reentering this facility after a discharge where return had not previously been expected. It is not completed following temporary discharges to hospitals or after therapeutic leaves/home visits.

MDS 2.0 10/18/94N   2 of 8   Produced using the Allu-Care LaserPrint System

Resident —————————— 07/31/1996 ————— Numeric Identifier —— 51-1166 ——————

MINIMUM DATA SET (MDS) - VERSION 2.0
FOR NURSING HOME RESIDENT ASSESSMENT AND CARE SCREENING
FULL ASSESSMENT FORM
(Status in last 7 days, unless other time frame indicated)

SECTION A. IDENTIFICATION INFORMATION

1.	RESIDENT NAME				
		a. (First)	b. (Middle Initial)	c. (Last)	d. (Jr./Sr.)

2.	ROOM NUMBER	4	2	0	B

3. ASSESSMENT REFERENCE DATE
a. Last day of MDS observation period

0	7		3	1		1	9	9	6
Month			Day			Year			

b. Original (0) or corrected copy of form (enter number of correction)

4a. DATE OF REENTRY
Date of reentry from most recent temporary discharge to a hospital in last 90 days (or since last assessment or admission if less than 90 days)

Month		Day		Year	

5.	MARITAL STATUS	1. Never married 3. Widowed 5. Divorced	
		2. Married 4. Separated	3

6.	MEDICAL RECORD NO.	5	·	1	-	1	1	6	6	·	·

7. CURRENT PAYMENT SOURCES FOR N.H. STAY
(Billing Office to indicate; check all that apply in last 30 days)

Medicaid per diem	a.	VA per diem	f.	
Medicare per diem	b.	Self or, family pays for full per diem	g.	X
Medicare ancillary part A	c.	Medicaid resident liability or Medicare co-payment	h.	
Medicare ancillary part B	d.	Private insurance per diem (including co-payment)	i.	
CHAMPUS per diem	e.	Other per diem	j.	

8. REASONS FOR ASSESSMENT
[Note-if this is a discharge or reentry assessment, only a limited subset of MDS items need be completed]

a. Primary reason for assessment
1. Admission assessment (required by day 14)
2. Annual assessment
3. Significant change in status assessment
4. Significant correction of prior assessment
5. Quarterly review assessment | 1
6. Discharged-return not anticipated
7. Discharged-return anticipated
8. Discharged prior to completing initial assessment
9. Reentry
0. NONE OF ABOVE

b. Special codes for use with supplemental assessment types in Case Mix demonstration states or other states where required
1. 5 day assessment
2. 30 day assessment
3. 60 day assessment
4. Quarterly assessment using full MDS form
5. Readmission/return assessment
6. Other state required assessment

9. RESPONSIBILITY/ LEGAL GUARDIAN
(Check all that apply)

Legal guardian	a. X	Durable power of attorney/ financial	d.
Other legal oversight	b.	Family member responsible	e.
Durable power of attorney/health care	c.	Patient responsible for self	f.
		NONE OF ABOVE	g.

10. ADVANCE DIRECTIVES
(For those items with supporting documentation in the medical record, check all that apply)

Living will	a.	Feeding restrictions	f.
Do not resuscitate	b.	Medication restrictions	g.
Do not hospitalize	c.	Other treatment restrictions	h.
Organ donation	d.		
Autopsy request	e.	NONE OF ABOVE	i. X

SECTION B. COGNITIVE PATTERNS   0

1.	COMATOSE	*(Persistent vegetative state/no discernible consciousness)*	
		0. No 1. Yes *(If yes, skip to Section G)*	0

2. MEMORY *(Recall of what was learned or known)*
a. Short-term memory OK - seems / appears to recall after 5 minutes
0. Memory OK   1. Memory problem 2 | 1

b. Long-term memory OK - seems / appears to recall long past
0. Memory OK   1. Memory problem 2 | 1

☐ = When box blank, must enter number or letter.

☐a = When letter in box, check if condition applies

Code "-" if information unavailable or unknown

MDS 2.0 10/18/94N

3 of 8

---

3. MEMORY / RECALL ABILITY
(Check all that resident was normally able to recall during last 7 days)

Current season	a.	That he/she is in a nursing home	d.
Location of own room	b.	NONE OF ABOVE are recalled	e.
Staff names / faces	c. X		

4. COGNITIVE SKILLS FOR DAILY DECISION-MAKING
(Made decisions regarding tasks of daily life)
0. INDEPENDENT - decisions consistent / reasonable
1. MODIFIED INDEPENDENCE - some difficulty in new situations only 2
2. MODERATELY IMPAIRED - decisions poor; cues/ supervision required 2
3. SEVERELY IMPAIRED - never/rarely made decisions 2, 5B | 3

5. INDICATORS OF DELIRIUM- PERIODIC DISORDERED THINKING/ AWARENESS
(Code for behavior in the last 7 days.) [Note: Accurate assessment requires conversations with staff and family who have direct knowledge of resident's behavior over this time.]
0. Behavior not present
1. Behavior present, not of recent onset
2. Behavior present, over last 7 days appears different from resident's usual functioning (e.g., new onset or worsening)

a. EASILY DISTRACTED - (e.g., difficulty paying attention; gets sidetracked) 2 = 1, 17* | 0

b. PERIODS OF ALTERED PERCEPTION OR AWARENESS OF SURROUNDINGS - (e.g., moves lips or talks to someone not present; believes he/she is somewhere else; confuses night and day) 2 = 1, 17* | 0

c. EPISODES OF DISORGANIZED SPEECH - (e.g., speech is incoherent, nonsensical, irrelevant, or rambling from subject to subject; loses train of thought) 2 = 1, 17* | 0

d. PERIODS OF RESTLESSNESS - (e.g., fidgeting or picking at skin,clothing,napkins, etc; frequent position changes;repetitive physical movements or calling out) 2 = 1, 17* | 0

e. PERIODS OF LETHARGY - (e.g., sluggishness; staring into space; difficult to arouse; little body movement) 2 = 1, 17* | 0

f. MENTAL FUNCTION VARIES OVER THE COURSE OF THE DAY - (e.g., sometimes better, sometimes worse; behaviors sometimes present, sometimes not) 2 = 1, 17* | 0

6. CHANGE IN COGNITIVE STATUS
Resident's cognitive status, skills, or abilities have changed as compared to status of 90 days ago or since assessment if less than 90 days)
0. No change   1. Improved   2. Deteriorated 1, 17* | 0

SECTION C. COMMUNICATION/HEARING PATTERNS

1. HEARING
(With hearing appliance, if used)
0. HEARS ADEQUATELY - normal talk, TV, phone
1. MINIMAL DIFFICULTY when not in quiet setting 4
2. HEARS IN SPECIAL SITUATIONS - speaker has to adjust tonal quality and speak distinctly 4
3. HIGHLY IMPAIRED / absence of useful hearing 4 | 3

2. COMMUNICATION DEVICES/ TECHNIQUES
(Check all that apply during last 7 days)

Hearing aid, present and used	a.
Hearing aid, present and not used regularly	b.
Other receptive comm. tecnniques used (e.g., lip reading)	c. X
NONE OF ABOVE	d.

3. MODES OF EXPRESSION
(Check all used by resident to make needs known)

Speech	a. X	Signs / gestures / sounds	d.
Writing messages to express or clarify	b.	Communication board	e.
American sign language or Braille	c.	Other	f.
		NONE OF ABOVE	g.

4. MAKING SELF UNDERSTOOD
(Expressing information content - however able)
0. UNDERSTOOD
1. USUALLY UNDERSTOOD - difficulty finding words or finishing thoughts 4
2. SOMETIMES UNDERSTOOD - ability is limited to making concrete requests 4
3. RARELY/NEVER UNDERSTOOD 4 | 1

5. SPEECH CLARITY
(Code for speech in the last 7 days)
0. CLEAR SPEECH - distinct, intelligible words
1. UNCLEAR SPEECH - slurred, mumbled words
2. NO SPEECH - absence of spoken words | 0

6. ABILITY TO UNDERSTAND OTHERS
(Understanding verbal information content - however able)
0. UNDERSTANDS
1. USUALLY UNDERSTANDS - may miss some part / intent of message 2, 4
2. SOMETIMES UNDERSTANDS - responds adequately to simple, direct communication 2, 4
3. RARELY/NEVER UNDERSTANDS 2, 4 | 2

7. CHANGE IN COMMUNICATION/ HEARING
Resident's ability to express, understand, or hear information has changed as compared to status of 90 days ago (or since last assessment if less than 90 days)
0. No change   1. Improved   2. Deteriorated 17* | 0

TRIGGER LEGEND
1 - Delirium
2 - Cognitive Loss / Dementia
4 - Communication
5B - ADL Maintenance
17* - Psychotropic Drugs
(For this to trigger, O4a, b, or c must = 1-7)

Resident _____

Numeric Identifier _____ 51-1166

SECTION D. VISION PATTERNS

1.	VISION	*(Ability to see in adequate light and with glasses if used)*
		0. *ADEQUATE* - sees fine detail, including regular print in newspapers / books
		1. *IMPAIRED* - sees large print, but not regular print in newspapers / books **3**
		2. *MODERATELY IMPAIRED* - limited vision: not able to see newspaper headlines, but can identify objects **1**
		3. *HIGHLY IMPAIRED* - object identification in question, but eyes appear to follow objects **3**
		4. *SEVERELY IMPAIRED* - no vision or sees only light, colors, or shapes; eyes do not appear to follow objects
2.	VISUAL LIMITATIONS/ DIFFICULTIES	Side vision problems - decreased peripheral vision (e.g., leaves food on one side of tray, difficulty traveling, bumps into people and objects, misjudges placement of chair when seating self) **3** a.
		Experiences any of following: sees halos or rings around lights; sees flashes of light; sees curtains over eyes b.
		NONE OF ABOVE c. **X**
3.	VISUAL APPLIANCES	Glasses; contact lenses; magnifying glass
		0. No 1. Yes **1**

SECTION E. MOOD AND BEHAVIOR PATTERNS

1.	INDICATORS OF DEPRES- SION, ANXIETY, SAD MOOD	*(Code for indicators observed in last 30 days, irrespective of the assumed cause)*
		0. Indicator not exhibited in last 30 days
		1. Indicator of this type exhibited up to five days a week
		2. Indicator of this type exhibited daily or almost daily (6, 7 days a week)

VERBAL EXPRESSIONS OF DISTRESS

a. Resident made negative statements - e.g., *"Nothing matters; Would rather be dead; What's the use; Regrets having lived so long; Let me die"* **1 or 2 = 8**	0	
b. Repetitive questions - e.g., *"Where do I go, What do I do?"* **1 or 2 = 8**	0	
c. Repetitive verbal- izations - e.g., calling out for help *("God help me")* **1 or 2 = 8**	0	
d. Persistent anger with self or others - e.g., easily annoyed, anger at placement in nursing home; anger at care received **1 or 2 = 8**	0	
e. Self depreciation - e.g., *"I am nothing; I am of no use to anyone"* **1 or 2 = 8**	0	
f. Expressions of what appear to be unreal- istic fears - e.g., fear of being abandoned, left alone, being with others **1 or 2 = 8**	0	
g. Recurrent statements that something terrible is about to happen - e.g., believes he or she is about to die, have a heart attack **1 or 2 = 8**	0	
h. Repetitive health complaints - e.g., persistently seeks medical attention, obsessive concern with body functions **1 or 2 = 8**	0	
i. Repetitive anxious complaints / concerns (non-health related) - e.g., persistently seeks attention / reassurance regarding schedules, meals, laundry/clothing, relationship issues **1 or 2 = 8**	0	

SLEEP-CYCLE ISSUES

j. Unpleasant mood in morning **1 or 2 = 8**	0	
k. Insomnia/change in usual sleep pattern **1 or 2 = 8**	0	

SAD, APATHETIC, ANXIOUS APPEARANCE

l. Sad, pained, worried facial expressions - e.g., furrowed brows **1 or 2 = 8**	0	
m. Crying, tearfulness **1 or 2 = 8**	0	
n. Repetitive physical movements - e.g., pacing, handwringing, restless- ness, fidgeting, picking **1 or 2 = 8, 17***	0	

LOSS OF INTEREST

o. Withdrawal from activities of interest - e.g., no interest in longstanding activities or being with family/ friends **1 or 2 = 7, 8**	0	
p. Reduced social inter- action **1 or 2 = 8**	0	

2.	MOOD PERSIS- TENCE	One or more indicators of depressed, sad or anxious mood were not easily altered by attempts to "cheer up", console, or reassure the resident over last 7 days
		0. No mood indicators 1. Indicators present, easily altered **8** 2. Indicators present, not easily altered **8** 0
3.	CHANGE IN MOOD	Resident's mood status has changed as compared to status of 90 days ago (or since last assessment if less than 90 days)
		0. No change 1. Improved 2. Deteriorated **1, 17*** 0
4.	BEHAVIORAL SYMPTOMS	*(A) Behavioral symptom frequency in last 7 days*
		0. Behavior not exhibited in last 7 days
		1. Behavior of this type occurred 1 to 3 days in last 7 days
		2. Behavior of this type occurred 4 to 6 days, but less than daily
		3. Behavior of this type occurred daily
		(B) Behavioral symptom alterability in last 7 days
		0. Behavior not present OR behavior was easily altered
		1. Behavior was not easily altered

	(A)	(B)
a. WANDERING (moved with no rational purpose, seemingly oblivious to needs or safety) **A = 1, 2, or 3 = 9, 11**	0	0
b. VERBALLY ABUSIVE BEHAVIORAL SYMPTOMS (others were threatened, screamed at, cursed at) **A = 1, 2, or 3 = 9**	0	0
c. PHYSICALLY ABUSIVE BEHAVIORAL SYMPTOMS (others were hit, shoved, scratched, sexually abused) **A = 1, 2 or 3 = 9**	0	0
d. SOCIALLY INAPPROPRIATE / DISRUPTIVE BEHAVIORAL SYMPTOMS (made disruptive sounds, noisiness, screaming, self-abusive acts, sexual behavior or disrobing in public, smeared/threw food/feces, hoarding, rummaged through other's belongings) **A = 1, 2, or 3 = 9**	0	0
e. RESISTS CARE (resisted taking medications/injections ADL assistance, or eating) **A = 1, 2, or 3 = 9**	0	0

SECTION F. PSYCHOSOCIAL WELL-BEING

5.	CHANGE IN BEHAVIORAL SYMPTOMS	Resident's behavior status has changed as compared to status of 90 days ago (or since last assessment if less than 90 days)
		0. No change 1. Improved **9** 2. Deteriorated **1, 17*** 0

1.	SENSE OF INITIATIVE/ INVOLVE- MENT	At ease interacting with others a.
		At ease doing planned or structured activities b.
		At ease doing self-initiated activities c.
		Establishes own goals **7** d.
		Pursues involvement in life of facility (e.g., makes/keeps friends; involved in group activities; responds positively to new activities; assists at religious services) e.
		Accepts invitations into most group activities f.
		NONE OF ABOVE g. **X**
2.	UNSETTLED RELATION- SHIPS	Covert/open conflict with or repeated criticism of staff **7** a.
		Unhappy with roommate **7** b.
		Unhappy with residents other than roommate **7** c.
		Openly expresses conflict/anger with family/friends **7** d.
		Absence of personal contact with family/friends e.
		Recent loss of close family member/friend f.
		Does not adjust easily to change in routines g.
		NONE OF ABOVE h. **X**
3.	PAST ROLES	Strong identification with past roles and life status **7** a.
		Expresses sadness/anger/empty feeling over lost roles / status **7** b.
		Resident perceives that daily routine (customary routine, activities) is very different from prior pattern in the community **7** c.
		NONE OF ABOVE d. **X**

SECTION G. PHYSICAL FUNCTIONING AND STRUCTURAL PROBLEMS

1.	(A) ADL SELF-PERFORMANCE - *(Code for resident's PERFORMANCE OVER ALL SHIFTS during last 7 days - Not including setup)*
		0. *INDEPENDENT* - NO help or oversight-OR-Help / oversight provided only **1 or 2** times during last 7 days
		1. *SUPERVISION* - Oversight, encouragement or cueing provided **3** or more times during last 7 days-OR-Supervision (3 or more times) plus physical assistance provided only **1 or 2** times during last 7 days
		2. *LIMITED ASSISTANCE* - Resident highly involved in activity; received physical help in guided maneuvering of limbs or other nonweight bearing assistance **3** or more times-OR-More help provided only **1 or 2** times during last 7 days
		3. *EXTENSIVE ASSISTANCE* - While resident performed part of activity, over last 7- day period, help of following type(s) provided **3** or more times: -Weight-bearing support -Full staff performance during part (but not all) of last 7 days
		4. *TOTAL DEPENDENCE* - Full staff performance of activity during entire 7 days
		8. *ACTIVITY DID NOT OCCUR* during entire 7 days

(B) ADL SUPPORT PROVIDED - *(Code for MOST SUPPORT PROVIDED OVER ALL SHIFTS during last 7 days; code regardless of resident's self-performance classification)*

0. No setup or physical help from staff   3. Two + persons physical assist
1. Setup help only   8. ADL activity itself did not
2. One person physical assist   occur during entire 7 days

			(A) SELF-PERF	(B) SUPPORT
a.	BED MOBILITY	How resident moves to and from lying position, turns side to side, and positions body while in bed **A = 1 = 5A; A = 2, 3, or 4 = 5A, 16; A = 8 = 16**	3	2
b.	TRANSFER	How resident moves between surfaces - to/from: bed, chair, wheelchair, standing position (EXCLUDE to/from bath/toilet) **A = 1, 2, 3, or 4 = 5A**	3	2
c.	WALK IN ROOM	How resident walks between locations in his/her room **A = 1, 2, 3, or 4 = 5A**	2	2
d.	WALK IN CORRIDOR	How resident walks in corridor on unit **A = 1, 2, 3, or 4 = 5A**	8	8
e.	LOCOMO- TION ON UNIT	How resident moves between locations in his/her room and adjacent corridor on same floor. If in wheelchair, self-sufficiency once in chair **A = 1, 2, 3, or 4 = 5A**	4	2
f.	LOCOMO- TION OFF UNIT	How resident moves to and returns from off unit locations (e.g., areas set aside for dining, activities, or treatments). If facility has only one floor, how resident moves to and from distant areas on the floor. If in wheelchair, self-sufficiency once in chair **A = 1, 2, 3, or 4 = 5A**	3	2
g.	DRESSING	How resident puts on, fastens, and takes off all items of street clothing, including donning/removing prosthesis **A = 1, 2, 3, or 4 = 5A**	3	2
h.	EATING	How resident eats and drinks (regardless of skill). Includes intake of nourishment by other means (e.g., tube feeding, total parenteral nutrition) **A = 1, 2, 3, or 4 = 5A**	3	2
i.	TOILET USE	How resident uses the toilet room (or commode, bedpan, urinal); transfers on/off toilet, cleanses, changes pad, manages ostomy or catheter, adjusts clothes **A = 1, 2, 3, or 4 = 5A**	4	2
j.	PERSONAL HYGIENE	How resident maintains personal hygiene, including combing hair, brushing teeth, shaving, applying makeup, washing/ drying face, hands, and perineum (EXCLUDE baths and showers) **A = 1, 2, 3, or 4 = 5A**	3	2

TRIGGER LEGEND

1 - Delirium
3 - Visual Function
5A - ADL Rehabilitation
7 - Psychosocial Well-being
8 - Mood State
9 - Behavior Symptoms
11 - Falls
17* - Psychotropic Drugs

(*For this to trigger, 04a, b. or c must = 1-7)

Resident _____ 07/31/1996 _____   Numeric Identifier ___ S1-1166 ___

2.	BATHING	How resident takes full-body bath/shower, sponge bath, and transfers in/out of tub/shower (EXCLUDE washing of back and hair). *Code for most dependent in self-performance and support. A = 1, 2, 3 or 4 = 5A* (A) BATHING SELF-PERFORMANCE codes appear below.	
		(A) (B)	
		0. Independent - No help provided	
		1. Supervision - Oversight help only	
		2. Physical help limited to transfer only	4 2
		3. Physical help in part of bathing activity	
		4. Total dependence	
		8. Activity itself did not occur during entire 7 days	
		(Bathing support codes are as defined in Item 1, code B above)	

3.	TEST FOR BALANCE (See training manual)	*(Code for ability during test in the last 7 days)* 0. Maintained position as required in test 1. Unsteady, but able to rebalance self without physical support 2. Partial physical support during test; or stands (sits) but does not follow directions for test 3. Not able to attempt test without physical help	
		a. Balance while standing	3
		b. Balance while sitting-position, trunk control 1, 2 or 3 = 17*	1

4.	FUNCTIONAL LIMITATION IN RANGE OF MOTION (see training manual)	*(Code for limitations during last 7 days that interfered with daily functions or placed resident at risk of injury)*		
		(A) RANGE OF MOTION (B) VOLUNTARY MOVEMENT		
		0. No limitation 0. No loss		
		1. Limitation on one side 1. Partial loss		
		2. Limitation on both sides 2. Full loss	(A)	(B)
		a. Neck	0	0
		b. Arm - including shoulder or elbow	0	0
		c. Hand - including wrist or fingers	0	0
		d. Leg - Including hip or knee	0	0
		e. Foot - Including ankle or toes	0	0
		f. Other limitation or loss	0	0

5.	MODES OF LOCOMOTION	*(Check all that apply during last 7 days)*			
		Cane/walker/crutch	a.	Wheelchair primary mode of locomotion	d. X
		Wheeled self	b.		
		Other person wheeled	c. X	NONE OF ABOVE	e.

6.	MODES OF TRANSFER	*(Check all that apply last 7 days)*			
		Bedfast all or most of time 16	a.	Lifted mechanically	d.
		Bed rails used for bed mobility or transfer	b.	Transfer aid (e.g., slide board, trapeze, cane, walker, brace)	e. X
		Lifted manually	c. X	NONE OF ABOVE	f.

7	TASK SEGMEN-TATION	Some or all of ADL activities were broken into subtasks during last 7 days so that resident could perform them	
		0. No 1. Yes	0

8.	ADL FUNCTIONAL REHABILITA-TION POTENTIAL	Resident believes he/she is capable of increased independence in at least some ADLs 5A	a.
		Direct care staff believe resident is capable of increased independence in at least some ADLs 5A	b.
		Resident able to perform tasks/activity but is very slow	c.
		Difference in ADL Self-Performance or ADL Support, comparing mornings to evenings	d.
		NONE OF ABOVE	e. X

9.	CHANGE IN ADL FUNCTION	Resident's ADL self-performance status has changed as compared to status of 90 days ago (or since last assessment if less than 90 days)	
		0. No change 1. Improved 2. Deteriorated	0

SECTION H. CONTINENCE IN LAST 14 DAYS

1.	CONTINENCE SELF-CONTROL CATEGORIES *(Code for resident's PERFORMANCE OVER ALL SHIFTS)*
	0. CONTINENT - Complete control *(includes use of indwelling urinary catheter or ostomy device that does not leak urine or stool)*
	1. USUALLY CONTINENT - BLADDER, incontinent episodes once a week or less; BOWEL, less than weekly
	2. OCCASIONALLY INCONTINENT - BLADDER, 2 or more times a week but not daily; BOWEL, once a week
	3. FREQUENTLY INCONTINENT - BLADDER, tended to be incontinent daily, but some control present (e.g., on day shift); BOWEL, 2-3 times a week
	4. INCONTINENT - Had inadequate control. BLADDER, multiple daily episodes; BOWEL, all (or almost all) of the time

a.	BOWEL CONTI-NENCE	Control of bowel movement, with appliance or bowel continence programs, if employed 1, 2, 3 or 4 = 16	4
b.	BLADDER CONTI-NENCE	Control of urinary bladder function (if dribbles, volume insufficient to soak through underpants), with appliances (e.g., foley) or continence programs, if employed 2, 3 or 4 = 6	4

2.	BOWEL ELIMIN-ATION PATTERN	Bowel elimination pattern regular-at least one movement every three days	a. X	Diarrhea	c.
		Constipation 17*	b.	Fecal impaction 17*	d.
				NONE OF ABOVE	e.

3.	APPLIANCES AND PROGRAMS	Any scheduled toileting plan	a. X	Did not use toilet room commode/urinal	f. X
		Bladder retraining program	b.	Pads/briefs used 6	g. X
		External (condom) catheter 6	c.	Enemas/irrigation	h.
		Indwelling catheter 6	d.	Ostomy present	i.
		Intermittent catheter 6	e.	NONE OF ABOVE	j.

4.	CHANGE IN URINARY CONTI-NENCE	Resident's urinary continence has changed as compared to status of 90 days ago (or since last assessment if less than 90 days)	
		0. No change 1. Improved 2. Deteriorated	0

SECTION I. DISEASE DIAGNOSES

Check only those diseases that have a relationship to current ADL status, cognitive status, mood and behavior status, medical treatments, nursing monitoring, or risk ot death. (Do not list inactive diagnoses)

1	DISEASES	*(If none apply, CHECK the NONE OF ABOVE box)*			
		ENDOCRINE/METABOLIC/ NUTRITIONAL		Hemiplegia / Hemiparesis	v.
		Diabetes mellitus	a.	Multiple sclerosis	w.
		Hyperthyroidism	b.	Paraplegia	x.
		Hypothyroidism	c.	Parkinson's disease	y.
		HEART/CIRCULATION		Quadriplegia	z.
		Arteriosclerotic heart disease (ASHD)	d.	Seizure disorder	aa.
		Cardiac dysrhythmias	e.	Transient ischemic attack (TIA)	bb.
		Congestive heart failure	f.	Traumatic brain injury	cc.
		Deep vein thrombosis	g.	PSYCHIATRIC/MOOD	
		Hypertension	h. X	Anxiety disorder	dd.
		Hypotension 17*	i.	Depression 17*	ee.
		Peripheral vascular disease	j.	Manic depression (bipolar disease)	ff.
		Other cardiovascular disease	k.	Schizophrenia	gg.
		MUSCULOSKELETAL		PULMONARY	
		Arthritis	l.	Asthma	hh.
		Hip fracture	m.	Emphysema/COPD	ii.
		Missing limb (e.g., amputation)	n.	SENSORY	
		Osteoporosis	o.	Cataracts 3	jj.
		Pathological bone fracture	p.	Diabetic retinopathy	kk.
		NEUROLOGICAL		Glaucoma 3	ll.
		Alzheimer's disease	q.	Macular degeneration	mm.
		Aphasia	r.	OTHER	
		Cerebral palsy	s.	Allergies	nn.
		Cerebrovascular accident (stroke)	t.	Anemia	oo. X
		Dementia other than Alzheimer's disease	u. X	Cancer	pp.
				Renal failure	qq.
				NONE OF ABOVE	rr.

2.	INFECTIONS	*(If none apply, CHECK the NONE OF ABOVE box)*			
		Antibiotic resistant infection (e.g., Methicillin resistant staph)	a.	Septicemia	g.
				Sexually transmitted diseases	h.
		Clostridium difficile (c. diff.)	b.	Tuberculosis	i.
		Conjunctivitis	c.	Urinary tract infection in last 30 days 14	j.
		HIV infection	d.	Viral hepatitis	k.
		Pneumonia	e.	Wound infection	l.
		Respiratory infection	f.	NONE OF ABOVE	m. X

3.	OTHER CURRENT OR MORE DETAILED DIAGNOSES AND ICD-9 CODES	Dehydration 276.5 = 14	a.	PROLAPSE W/O VAGINAL WALL	≤18 • 1
			b.	CLSD FX PART NK FEM NOS	E20 • 8
			c.	FX PELV CLSD NOS	808 • 8
			d.		•
			e.		•

SECTON J. HEALTH CONDITIONS

1.	PROBLEM CONDITIONS	*(Check all problems present in last 7 days unless other time frame is indicated)*			
		INDICATORS OF FLUID STATUS		Dizziness/Vertigo 11,17*	f.
		Weight gain or loss of 3 or more pounds within a 7 day period 14	a.	Edema	g.
				Fever 14	h.
		Inability to lie flat due to shortness of breath	b.	Hallucinations 17*	i.
		Dehydrated; output exceeds input 14	c.	Internal bleeding 14	j.
				Recurrent lung aspirations in last 90 days 17*	k.
		Insufficient fluid; did NOT consume all/almost all liquids provided during last 3 days 14	d.	Shortness of breath	l.
				Syncope (fainting) 17*	m.
		OTHER		Unsteady gait 17*	n. X
		Delusions	e.	Vomiting	o.
				NONE OF ABOVE	p.

‐GER LEGEND
3 - Visual Function
5A - ADL Rehabilitation
6 - Urinary Incontinence / Indwelling Catheter
11 - Falls

14 - Dehydration/Fluid Maintenance
16 - Pressure Ulcers
17* - Psychotropic Drugs
(*For this to trigger. 04a. b, or c must = 1-7)

MDS 2.0 10/18/94N   5 of 8

07/31/1996   51-1166

Resident _____   Numeric Identifier _____

2.	PAIN SYMPTOMS	*(Code the highest level of pain present in the last 7 days)*		
		a. FREQUENCY with which resident complains or shows evidence of pain	b. INTENSITY of pain	
		0. No pain *(skip to J4)*	1. Mild pain	
		1. Pain less than daily	2. Moderate pain	
		2. Pain daily	3. Times when pain is horrible or excruciating	
		0		

3.	PAIN SITE	*(If pain present, check all sites that apply in last 7 days)*		
		Back pain	a.	Incisional pain	f.
		Bone pain	b.	Joint pain (other than hip)	g.
		Chest pain while doing usual activities	c.	Soft tissue pain (e.g., lesion, muscle)	h.
		Headache	d.	Stomach pain	i.
		Hip pain	e.	Other	j.

4.	ACCIDENTS	(Check all that apply).	
		Fell in past 30 days 11, 17*	a.	Hip fracture in last 180 days 17*	c.
		Fell in past 31-180 days 11, 17*	b.	Other fracture in last 180 days	d.
				NONE OF ABOVE	e. X

5.	STABILITY OF CONDITIONS	Conditions/diseases make resident's cognitive, ADL, mood or behavior patterns unstable - (fluctuating, precarious, or deteriorating)	a.
		Resident experiencing an acute episode or a flare-up of a recurrent or chronic problem	b.
		End-stage disease, 6 or fewer months to live	c.
		NONE OF ABOVE	d. X

SECTION K. ORAL/NUTRITIONAL STATUS

1.	ORAL PROBLEMS	Chewing problem	a. X
		Swallowing problem 17*	b.
		Mouth pain 15	c.
		NONE OF ABOVE	d.

2.	HEIGHT AND WEIGHT	*Record (a.) height in inches and (b.) weight in pounds. Base weight on most recent measure in last 30 days; measure weight consistently in accord with standard facility practice - e.g., in a.m. after voiding, before meal, with shoes off, and in nightclothes.*				
		a. HT (in.)	6	1	b. WT (lb.)	9	7

3.	WEIGHT CHANGE	a. Weight loss - 5% or more in last 30 days; or 10% or more in last 180 days	
		0. No 1. Yes 12	0
		b. Weight gain - 5% or more in last 30 days; or 10% or more in last 180 days	
		0. No 1. Yes	0

4.	NUTRITIONAL PROBLEMS	Complains about the taste of many foods 12	a.	Leaves 25% or more of food uneaten at most meals 12	c. X
		Regular or repetitive complaints of hunger	b.	NONE OF ABOVE	d.

5.	NUTRITIONAL APPROACHES	*(Check all that apply in last 7 days)*			
		Parenteral / IV 12, 14	a.	Dietary supplement between meals	f. X
		Feeding tube 12, 14	b.	Plate guard, stabilized built-up utensil, etc.	g.
		Mechanically altered diet 12	c. X	On a planned weight change program	h.
		Syringe (oral feeding) 12	d.	NONE OF ABOVE	i.
		Therapeutic diet 12	e.		

6.	PARENTERAL OR ENTERAL INTAKE	a. *(Skip to Section L if neither 5a nor 5b is checked)* Code the proportion of total calories the resident received through parenteral or tube feedings in the last 7 days	
		0. None 3. 51 % to 75%	
		1. 1% to 25% 4. 76% to 100%	
		2. 26% to 50%	
		b. Code the average fluid intake per day by IV or tube in last 7 days	
		0. None 3. 1001 to 1500 cc/day	
		1. 1 to 500 cc/day 4. 1501 to 2000 cc/day	
		2. 501 to 1000 cc/day 5. 2001 or more cc/day	

SECTION L. ORAL/DENTAL STATUS

1.	ORAL STATUS AND DISEASE PREVENTION	Debris (soft, easily movable substances) present in mouth prior to going to bed at night 15	a.
		Has dentures or removable bridge	b. X
		Some/all natural teeth lost - does not have or does not use dentures (or partial plates) 15	c.
		Broken, loose, or carious teeth 15	d.
		Inflamed gums (gingiva); swollen or bleeding gums; oral abscesses; ulcers or rashes 15	e.
		Daily cleaning of teeth/dentures or daily mouth care - by resident or staff Not / = 15	f. X
		NONE OF ABOVE	g.

SECTION M. SKIN CONDITION

1.	ULCERS (Due to any cause)	*(Record the number of ulcers at each ulcer stage - regardless of cause. If none present at a stage, record "0" (zero). Code all that apply during last 7 days. Code 9 = 9 or more.) [Requires full body exam.]*	Number at Stage
		a. Stage 1. A persistent area of skin redness (without a break in the skin) that does not disappear when pressure is relieved.	0
		b. Stage 2. A partial thickness loss of skin layers that presents clinically as an abrasion, blister, or shallow crater.	0
		c. Stage 3. A full thickness of skin is lost, exposing the sub-cutaneous tissues-presents as a deep crater with or without undermining adjacent tissue.	0
		d. Stage 4. A full thickness of skin and subcutaneous tissue is lost, exposing muscle or bone.	0

2.	TYPE OF ULCER	*(For each type of ulcer, code for the highest stage in the last 7 days using scale in item M1 - i.e., 0 = none; stages 1, 2, 3, 4)*	
		a. Pressure ulcer-any lesion caused by pressure resulting in damage of underlying tissue 1 = 16; 2, 3, or 4 = 12, 16	0
		b. Stasis ulcer-open lesion caused by poor circulation in the lower extremities	0

3.	HISTORY OF RESOLVED ULCERS	Resident had an ulcer that was resolved or cured in LAST 90 DAYS	
		0. No 1. Yes 16	0

4.	OTHER SKIN PROBLEMS OR LESIONS PRESENT	*(Check all that apply during last 7 days)*	
		Abrasions, bruises	a.
		Burns (second or third degree)	b.
		Open lesions other than ulcers, rashes, cuts (e.g., cancer lesions)	c.
		Rashes - e.g., intertrigo, eczema, drug rash, heat rash, herpes zoster	d.
		Skin desensitized to pain or pressure 16	e. X
		Skin tears or cuts (other than surgery)	f.
		Surgical wounds	g.
		NONE OF ABOVE	h.

5.	SKIN TREATMENTS	*(Check all that apply during last 7 days)*	
		Pressure relieving device(s) for chair	a. X
		Pressure relieving device(s) for bed	b. X
		Turning/repositioning program	c. X
		Nutrition or hydration intervention to manage skin problems	d.
		Ulcer care	e.
		Surgical wound care	f.
		Application of dressings (with or without topical medications) other than to feet	g.
		Application of ointments/medications (other than to feet)	h.
		Other preventative or protective skin care (other than to feet)	i.
		NONE OF ABOVE	j.

6.	FOOT PROBLEMS AND CARE	*(Check all that apply during last 7 days)*	
		Resident has one or more foot problems (e.g., corns, calluses, bunions, hammer toes, overlapping toes, pain, structural problems	a.
		Infection of the foot - e.g., cellulitis, purulent drainage	b.
		Open lesions on the foot	c.
		Nails/calluses trimmed during last 90 days	d. X
		Received preventative or protective foot care (e.g., used special shoes, inserts, pads, toe separators)	e.
		Application of dressings (with or without topical medications)	f.
		NONE OF ABOVE	g.

SECTION N. ACTIVITY PURSUIT PATTERNS

1.	TIME AWAKE	*(Check appropriate time periods over last 7 days)* Resident awake all or most of time (i.e., naps no more than one hour per time period) in the:	
	10B only if BOTH N 1a = 3nd N2 = 0	Morning 10B	a. X	Evening	c.
		Afternoon	b.	NONE OF ABOVE	d.

(IF RESIDENT IS COMATOSE, SKIP TO SECTION O)

2.	AVERAGE TIME INVOLVED IN ACTIVITIES	*(When awake and not receiving treatments or ADL care)*	
		0. Most - more than 2/3 of time 10B 2. Little - less than 1/3 of time 10A	
		1. Some - from 1/3 to 2/3 of time 3. None 10A	1

3.	PREFERRED ACTIVITY SETTINGS	*(Check all settings in which activities are preferred)*	
		Own room	a. X		
		Day/activity room	b.	Outside facility	d.
		Inside NH/off unit	c.	NONE OF ABOVE	e.

4.	GENERAL ACTIVITY PREFERENCES (Adapted to resident's current abilities)	*(Check all PREFERENCES whether or not activity is currently available to resident)*	
		Cards/other games	a.	Trips / shopping	g.
		Crafts/arts	b.	Walking / wheeling outdoors	h.
		Exercise/sports	c.	Watching TV	i.
		Music	d. X	Gardening or plants	j.
		Reading/writing	e.	Talking or conversing	k. X
		Spiritual/religious activities	f.	Helping others	l.
				NONE OF ABOVE	m.

GGER LEGEND
10A - Activities (Revise)   13 - Feeding Tubes   17* - Psychotropic Drugs
10B - Activities (Review)   14 - Dehydration/ Fluid Maintenance   (*For this to trigger, 04a, b, or c must = 1-7)
11 - Falls   15 - Dental Care
12 - Nutritional Status   16 - Pressure Ulcers

MDS 2.0 10/18/94N   6 of 8

Resident _____ 07/31/1996 _____ Numeric Identifier __51-1166__

5.	PREFERS CHANGE IN DAILY ROUTINE	Code for resident preferences in daily routines 0. No change 1. Slight change 2. Major change		
		a. Type of activities in which resident is currently involved 1 or 2 = 10A	0	
		b. Extent of resident involvement in activities 1 or 2 = 10A	0	

SECTION O. MEDICATIONS

1.	NUMBER OF MEDICATIONS	(Record the number of different medications used in the last 7 days; enter "0" if none used)		03
2.	NEW MEDICA-TIONS	(Resident currently receiving medications that were initiated during the last 90 days) 0. No 1. Yes		0
3.	INJECTIONS	(Record the number of DAYS injections of any type received during the last 7 days; enter "0" if none used)		0
4.	DAYS RECEIVED THE FOLLOWING MEDICATION	(Record the number of DAYS during last 7 days; enter "0" if not used. Note - enter "1" for long-acting meds used less than weekly) (NOTE: For 17 to actually be triggered, 04a, b, or c MUST = 1-7 AND at least one additional item marked 17* must be indicated. See sections B, C, D, H, I, J, and K.)		

	a. Antipsychotic 1-7 = 17	0	d. Hypnotic	0
	b. Antianxiety 1-7 = 11,17	0	e. Diuretic 1-7 = 14	0
	c. Antidepressant 1-7 = 11,17	0		

SECTION P. SPECIAL TREATMENTS AND PROCEDURES

1.	SPECIAL TREAT-MENTS, PROCE-DURES, AND PROGRAMS	a. SPECIAL CARE - Check treatments received during the last 14 days [Note - count only post admission treatments]

TREATMENTS			PROGRAMS		
Chemotherapy	a.		Ventilator or respirator	l.	
Dialysis	b.		Alcohol/drug treatment program	m.	
IV medication	c.		Alzheimer's/dementia special care unit	n.	
Intake / output	d.		Hospice care	o.	
Monitoring acute medical condition	e.		Pediatric unit	p.	
Ostomy care	f.		Respite care	q.	
Oxygen therapy	g.		Training in skills required to return to the community (e.g., taking medications, house work, shopping, transportation, ADLs)	r.	
Radiation	h.				
Suctioning	i.				
Tracheostomy care	j.				
Transfusions	k.		NONE OF ABOVE	s.	X

b. THERAPIES - Record the number of days and total minutes each of the following therapies were administered (for at least 15 minutes a day) in the last 7 calendar days [Enter 0 if none or less than 15 min daily] [Note - count only post admission therapies]

(A) = # of days administered for 15 minutes or more
(B) = total # of minutes provided in last 7 days

	DAYS (A)	MIN (B)
a. Speech-language pathology and audiology services	0	0000
b. Occupational therapy	0	0000
c. Physical therapy	0	0000
d. Respiratory therapy	0	0000
e. Psychological therapy (by any licensed mental health professional)	0	0000

2.	INTERVEN-TION PROGRAMS FOR MOOD, BEHAVIOR, COGNITIVE LOSS	(Check all interventions or strategies used in last 7 days - no matter where received)		
		Special behavior symptom evaluation program	a.	
		Evaluation by a licensed mental health specialist in last 90 days	b.	X
		Group therapy	c.	
		Resident - specific deliberate changes in the environment to address mood / behavior patterns - e.g., providing bureau in which to rummage	d.	
		Reorientation - e.g., cueing	e.	X
		NONE OF ABOVE	f.	

3.	NURSING REHABILI-TATION/ RESTOR-ATIVE CARE	Record the NUMBER OF DAYS each of the following rehabilitation or restorative techniques or practices was provided to the resident for more than or equal to 15 minutes per day in the last 7 days (Enter 0 if none or less than 15 min. daily.)		
		a. Range of motion (passive)		f. Walking	0
		b. Range of motion (active)	7 / 0	g. Dressing or grooming	0
		c. Splint or brace assistance	0	h. Eating or swallowing	0
		TRAINING AND SKILL PRACTICE IN:		i. Amputation/ prosthesis care	0
		d. Bed mobility	0	j. Communication	0
		e. Transfer	0	k. Other	0

4.	DEVICES AND RESTRAINTS	(Use the following codes for last 7 days:) 0. Not used 1. Used less than daily 2. Used daily		
		Bed rails		
		a. - Full bed rails on all open sides of bed	2	
		b. - Other types of side rails used (e.g., half rail, one side)	0	
		c. Trunk restraint 1 = 11, 18; 2 = 11, 16, 18	0	
		d. Limb restraint 1 or 2 = 18	0	
		e. Chair prevents rising 1 or 2 = 18	0	
5.	HOSPITAL STAY(S)	Record number of times resident was admitted to hospital with an overnight stay in last 90 days (or since last assessment if less than 90 days). (Enter 0 if no hospital admissions)		00
6.	EMERGENCY ROOM (ER) VISIT(G)	Record number of times resident visited ER without an overnight stay in last 90 days (or since last assessment if less than 90 days). (Enter 0 if no ER visits)		00
7.	PHYSICIAN VISITS	In the LAST 14 DAYS (or since admission if less than 14 days in facility) how many days has the physician (or authorized assistant or practitioner) examined the resident? (Enter 0 if none)		01
8.	PHYSICIAN ORDERS	In the LAST 14 DAYS (or since admission if less than 14 days in facility) how many days has the physician (or authorized assistant or practitioner) changed the resident's orders? Do not include order renewals without change. (Enter 0 if none)		01
9.	ABNORMAL LAB VALUES	Has the resident had any abnormal lab values during the last 90 days (or since admission)? 0. No 1. Yes		0

SECTION Q. DISCHARGE POTENTIAL AND OVERALL STATUS

1.	DISCHARGE POTENTIAL	a. Resident expresses/indicates preference to return to the community 0. No 1. Yes	0
		b. Resident has a support person who is positive toward discharge 0. No 1. Yes	0
		c. Stay projected to be of a short duration-discharge projected within 90 days (do not include expected discharge due to death) 0. No 2. Within 31 - 90 days 1. Within 30 days 3. Discharge status uncertain	0
2.	OVERALL CHANGE IN CARE NEEDS	Resident's overall self sufficiency has changed significantly as compared to status of 90 days ago (or since last assessment if less than 90 days) 0. No change 1. Improved - receives fewer supports, needs less restrictive level of care 2. Deteriorated - receives more support	0

SECTION R. ASSESSMENT INFORMATION

1.	PARTICI-PATION IN ASSESSMENT	a. Resident:	0. No	1. Yes		0
		b. Family:	0. No	1. Yes	2. No family	1
		c. Significant other:	0. No	1. Yes	2. None	0

2. SIGNATURES OF PERSONS COMPLETING THE ASSESSMENT:

a. Signature of RN Assessment Coordinator (sign on above line)

b. Date RN Assessment Coordinator signed as complete

	0	7	—	3	1	—	1	9	9	7
		Month		Day				Year		

c. Other Signatures	Title	Sections	Date
d.			Date
e.			Date
f.			Date
g.			Date
h.			Date

TRIGGER LEGEND
10A - Activities (Revise)   16 - Pressure Ulcers
11 - Falls   17 - Psychotropic Drugs
4 - Dehydration/Fluid Maintenance   18 - Physical Restraints

07/31/1996

SECTION V. RESIDENT ASSESSMENT PROTOCOL SUMMARY   51-1166

Numeric Identifier

Resident's Name: **John Doe**

Medical Record No.:

Check if RAP is triggered.

2. For each triggered RAP, use the RAP guidelines to identify areas needing further assessment. Document relevant assessment information regarding the resident's status.

- Describe:
  - Nature of the condition (may include presence or lack of objective data and subjective complaints).
  - Complications and risk factors that affect your decision to proceed to care planning.
  - Factors that must be considered in developing individualized care plan interventions.
  - Need for referrals/further evaluation by appropriate health professionals.

- Documentation should support your decision-making regarding whether to proceed with a care plan for a triggered RAP and the type(s) of care plan interventions that are appropriate for a particular resident.

- Documentation may appear anywhere in the clinical record (e.g., progress notes, consults, flowsheets, etc.).

3. Indicate under the Location of RAP Assessment Documentation column where information related to the RAP assessment can be found.

4. For each triggered RAP, indicate whether a new care plan, care plan revision, or continuation of current care plan is necessary to address the problem(s) identified in your assessment. The Care Planning Decision column must be completed within 7 days of completing the RAI (MDS and RAPs).

A. RAP Problem Area	(a) Check if Triggered	Location and Date of RAP Assessment Documentation	(b) Care Planning Decision-check if addressed in care plan
1. DELIRIUM			
2. COGNITIVE LOSS	x	RAP 2 7/30/96	✓
3. VISUAL FUNCTION	x	RAP 3 "	
4. COMMUNICATION	x	RAP 4 "	
5. ADL FUNCTIONAL / REHABILITATION POTENTIAL	x	RAP 5 "	✓
URINARY INCONTINENCE AND INDWELLING CATHETER	x	RAP 6 "	✓
7. PSYCHOSOCIAL WELL-BEING			
8. MOOD STATE			
9. BEHAVIORAL SYMPTOMS			
10. ACTIVITIES			
11. FALLS	x	RAP 11 7/30/96	✓
12. NUTRITIONAL STATUS	x	RAP 12 7/29/96	✓
13. FEEDING TUBES			
14. DEHYDRATION/FLUID MAINTENANCE	✓	RAP 14 7/30/96	
15. ORAL/DENTAL CARE			
16. PRESSURE ULCERS	x	RAP 16 7/30/96	
17. PSYCHOTROPIC DRUG USE	x	RAP 17 7/30/96	
18. PHYSICAL RESTRAINTS			

B. *John Doe*

1. Signature of RN Coordinator for RAP Assessment Process

2. 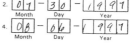
| 0 | 7 | – | 3 | 0 | – | 1 | 9 | 9 | 7 |
Month   Day   Year

3. Signature of Person Completing Care Planning Decision

4.
| 0 | 8 | – | 0 | 6 | – | 1 | 9 | 9 | 7 |
Month   Day   Year

APPENDIX **D**

NANDA-Approved Nursing Diagnoses (through 12th NANDA Conference)†

Activity Intolerance
Activity Intolerance, Risk for
Adaptive Capacity: Intracranial, Decreased
Adjustment, Impaired
Airway Clearance, Ineffective
Anxiety [specify level]*
Aspiration, Risk for
Body Image Disturbance
Body Temperature, Risk for Altered
Bowel Incontinence
Breastfeeding, Effective
Breastfeeding, Ineffective
Breastfeeding, Interrupted
Breathing Pattern, Ineffective
Cardiac Output, Decreased
Caregiver Role Strain
Caregiver Role Strain, Risk for
Communication, Impaired Verbal
Community Coping, Ineffective
Community Coping, Potential for Enhanced
Confusion, Acute
Confusion, Chronic
Constipation
Constipation, Colonic
Constipation, Perceived

Coping, Defensive
Coping, Individual, Ineffective
Decisional Conflict (Specify)
Denial, Ineffective
Diarrhea
Disuse Syndrome, Risk for
Diversional Activity Deficit
Dysreflexia
Energy Field Disturbance
Environmental Interpretation Syndrome,
  Impaired
Family Coping: Compromised, Ineffective
Family Coping: Disabling, Ineffective
Family Coping: Potential for Growth
Family Process: Alcoholism, Altered
Family Processes, Altered
Fatigue
Fear
Fluid Volume Deficit [active loss]*
Fluid Volume Deficit [regulatory failure]*
Fluid Volume Deficit, Risk for
Fluid Volume Excess

(table continues)

†Permission from North American Nursing Diagnosis Association (1997). NANDA Nursing Diagnoses: Definitions and Classifications 1997–1998. Philadelphia. NANDA. Copyright 1996 by the North American Nursing Diagnosis Association.

Gas Exchange, Impaired
Grieving, Anticipatory
Grieving, Dysfunctional
Growth and Development, Altered
Health Maintenance, Altered
Health-Seeking Behaviors (Specify)
Home Maintenance Management, Impaired
Hopelessness
Hyperthermia
Hypothermia
Incontinence, Functional
Incontinence, Reflex
Incontinence, Stress
Incontinence, Total
Incontinence, Urge
Infant Behavior, Disorganized
Infant Behavior, Disorganized, Risk for
Infant Behavior, Organized, Potential for
  Enhanced
Infant Feeding Pattern, Ineffective
Infection, Risk for
Injury, Risk for
Knowledge Deficit [learning need]* (Specify)
Loneliness, Risk for
Memory, Impaired
Noncompliance [Compliance, altered]* (specify)
Nutrition: Less than Body Requirements, Altered
Nutrition: More than Body Requirements,
  Altered
Nutrition: Potential for More than Body
  Requirements, Altered
Oral Mucous Membrane, Altered
Pain [acute]
Pain, Chronic
Parent/Infant/Child Attachment, Risk for Altered
Parental Role Conflict
Parenting, Altered
Parenting, Risk for Altered
Perioperative Positioning Injury, Risk for
Peripheral Neurovascular Dysfunction, Risk for
Personal Identity Disturbance
Physical Mobility, Impaired
Poisoning, Risk for
Post-Trauma Response
Powerlessness
Protection, Altered
Rape-Trauma Syndrome
Rape-Trauma Syndrome: Compound Reaction

Rape-Trauma Syndrome: Silent Reaction
Relocation Stress Syndrome
Role Performance, Altered
Self Care Deficit, Bathing/Hygiene,
  Dressing/Feeding, Grooming, Toileting
Self Esteem, Chronic Low
Self Esteem Disturbance
Self Esteem, Situational Low
Self-Mutilation, Risk for
Sensory/Perceptual Alterations (Specify): visual,
  auditory, kinesthetic, gustatory, tactile,
  olfactory
Sexual Dysfunction
Sexuality Patterns, Altered
Skin Integrity, Impaired
Skin Integrity Risk for Impaired
Sleep Pattern Disturbance
Social Interaction, Impaired
Social Isolation
Spiritual Distress (distress of the human spirit)
Spiritual Well-Being, Potential for Enhanced
Spontaneous Ventilation, Inability to Sustain
Suffocation, Risk for
Swallowing, Impaired
Therapeutic Regimen: Community, Ineffective
  Management
Therapeutic Regimen: Families, Ineffective
  Management
Therapeutic Regimen: Individuals, Effective
  Management
Therapeutic Regimen (Individuals), Ineffective
  Management
Thermoregulation, Ineffective
Thought Processes, Altered
Tissue Integrity, Impaired
Tissue Perfusion, Altered (Specify Type):
  cerebral, cardiopulmonary, renal,
  gastrointestinal, peripheral
Trauma, Risk for
Unilateral Neglect
Urinary Elimination, Altered
Urinary Retention [acute/chronic]*
Ventilatory Weaning Response, Dysfunctional
  (DVWR)
Violence, Risk for: Self directed or directed at
  others

---

* [Author recommendations]

APPENDIX E

Use of Complementary Therapies in Long Term Care

Complementary therapies, sometimes referred to as alternative medicine or enhancement therapy, allow residents to integrate the mind, body, and spirit, while becoming active participants in healing and health care. Although not an alternative to traditional medicine, complementary therapies augment the effects of surgery, drugs, and other medical treatments.

The use of complementary therapies is a growing trend in the United States. Recent studies indicate that more dollars are spent on these therapies than on conventional medicine (Eisenberg et al, 1993; Paramore, 1997).

Nurses, physicians, and other health care professionals throughout the country are using complementary therapies as part of their practices. This appendix briefly describes some of the common, low-risk modalities that may be used in long term care settings, including prayer, relaxation, imagery, music, touch, and humor.

Prayer

Prayer is related to religion and spirituality. Research has demonstrated that when adults undergo a crisis or life-threatening event, spirituality and religion become very important (Camp, 1996).

Although prayer has many forms and expressions, it can be generally defined as "a representation of one's longing for communion or communication with God or the Absolute" (Dossey, 1997, p. 45). In collaboration with the social worker and activity therapist, the long term care nurse can elp residents reflect on the meaning of prayer and religion in their lives. Some residents enjoy inspirational readings, religious music, and church services.

Relaxation

Relaxation is one of the easiest techniques to learn and one of the most beneficial for the resident. Relaxation has many positive physiologic effects, as well as psychosocial outcomes. Some examples of physiologic changes include decreased blood pressure, increased peripheral blood flow, and increased activity of immune killer cells that fight infection. The simplest relaxation modality is progressive muscle relaxation (PMR).

PMR is based on the fact that stress increases skeletal muscle tension. Intentional tensing and releasing of successive muscle groups decreases anxiety and promotes relaxation. To begin PMR, the nurse asks the resident to take several deep breaths with eyes closed. Then the resident tenses and releases each muscle group for several seconds, starting with the head, and progressing to the toes. Richards (1996) found that caring interventions that focus on the body-mind connection, such as muscle relaxation, back rubs, and music, promote sleep in the elderly.

Imagery

Imagery is a technique by which a person experiences dreams, visions, and memories as a way of making the mind-body-spirit connection. Images can be induced or may occur spontaneously. Although all senses may be involved, most images are visual in that the individual sees positive mental pictures, such as mountains or sunsets.

Imagery produces physiologic effects that affect healing. In particular, imagery increases production of neurotransmitters (norepinephrine and acetylcholine) in the brain that promote relaxation.

Music

Music also stimulates the autonomic, immune, and endocrine systems to help relax residents, thereby reducing anxiety, pain, and stress. For elderly residents who are confused and restless, Ragneskog et al (1996) found that the calming effect of music improved behavioral manifestations such as agitation and combativeness.

In collaboration with the activity therapist, the nurse selects music that is soothing and reminds clients of the past. Music creates a variety of experiences for the client, including imagery and sensory stimulation.

Touch

The use of various forms of touch has been documented for more than 5000 years. Touch slows the heart, decreases diastolic blood pressure, and reduces anxiety. Research has shown that older residents are likely to receive the least amount of touch, and yet they need touch as much as, if not more than, any other age group (Dossey et al, 1995). However, severely agitated elderly residents may not want to be touched because they may view touch as an invasion of their personal space.

Some of the most common forms of touch therapy include therapeutic massage, acupressure, reflexology, and therapeutic touch. All of these techniques require specialized training, yet the back rub is a type of therapeutic massage that nurses have been administering for most of the 20th century. Back rubs and massage can promote relaxation and sleep, as well as provide a distraction for the resident experiencing pain or anxiety.

Laughter and Humor

Like the other modalities, laughter and humor have positive effects on the immune, cardiovascular, and endocrine systems. The psychologic effects result in stress reduction, distraction, and relaxation. People who have a strong sense of humor generally deal better with stress than those who do not.

Nurses often use laughter and humor as part of their daily resident care. Some long term care agencies have mobile comedy carts, humor areas, or clown visitation programs. All of these activities help distract the resident, relieve pain, and promote stress relief.

REFERENCES

Camp, P. E. (1996). Having faith: Experiencing coronary artery bypass grafting. *Journal of Cardiovascular Nursing, 10*(3), 55–64.
Dossey, B. M. (1997). *Core curriculum for holistic nursing.* Gaithersburg, MD: Aspen.
Dossey, B. M., Keegan, L., Guzzetta, C. E., and Kolkmeir, L. G. (1995). *Holistic nursing: A handbook for practice.* Gaithersburg, MD: Aspen.
Eisenberg, D. M., Kessler, R. C., Foster, C. et al (1993). Unconventional medicine in the United States—Prevalence, costs, and patterns of use. *New England Journal of Medicine, 328*, 246–252.
Paramore, L. C. (1997). Use of alternative therapies: Estimates from the 1994 Robert Wood Johnson Foundation National Access to Care Survey. *Journal of Pain and Symptom Management, 13*(2), 83–89.
Ragneskog, H., Kihlgren, M., Karlsson, I., and Norberg, A. (1996). Dinner music for demented patients: Analysis of video-recorded observations. *Clinical Nursing Research, 5*(3), 262–277.
Richards, K. C. (1996). Sleep promotion. *Critical Care Clinics of North America, 8*(1), 39–52.

APPENDIX F

Operational Standards for Medication Pass

- The facility has a mechanism for recording and reporting medication errors.
- The facility calculates and monitors its medication error rate.
- The facility takes corrective action when significant medication errors are noted.
- The facility takes disciplinary action against employees who repeatedly make medication errors.
- The facility is free of any omitted administration of any cardiovascular drug.
- The facility is free of any unauthorized administration of any diuretic or cardiovascular or antipsychotic drug.
- The facility is free of any wrong dose of digoxin or dilantin being administered.
- The facility is free from having any eye drop being administered in the wrong eye.
- All antibiotics have been administered in relationship to meals.
- All residents receiving anticonvulsants, anticoagulants, antiarrhythmic, antianginal, and antiglaucoma drugs have evidence that their blood levels of these drugs are titrated.
- Residents are free from adverse effects associated with medication errors.

Index

AARP. *See* American Association of Retired Persons

ABCD rule, 151

Abnormal involuntary movement scale (AIMS), 68

Accommodation, 192

Accreditation, 17–18, 203

Accupril, 117

ACE inhibitor. *See* Angiotensin converting enzyme (ACE) inhibitor

Acetaminophen, 89, 98

ACLS. *See* Advanced Certification in Life Support

Acquired immunodeficiency syndrome. *See* AIDS

ACS. *See* American Cancer Society

Activated partial thromboplastin time (APTT), 127

Activities of daily living (ADLs), 11, 34, 62, 171, 173

Activity therapy, 173

Activity/treatment record, 143

Acute infection(s), 108–12

Acute pain, 95–96, 97t

Acute peripheral vascular occlusion, 126–28, 127t

Acute urinary incontinence, 52

ADA. *See* American Diabetes Association

ADLs. *See* Activities of daily living

Administrator-in-training (AIT), 167

Admissions, 33–34

ADN/ADON. *See* Assistant director of nursing

Advanced Certification in Life Support (ACLS), 157

Advanced directives, 218–19

Advil, 89

Agency for Health Care Policy and Research (AHCPR), 45, 49, 58

Aging
demographics of, 2–3
laboratory tests and, 27–29, 27t, 35
physiologic changes with, 22–27, 35
psychosocial changes with, 29–31, 35
See also Elderly

AHCA. *See* American Health Care Association

AHCPR. *See* Agency for Health Care Policy and Research

AIDS (acquired immunodeficiency syndrome)
dementia and, 59
See also HIV

AIMS. *See* Abnormal involuntary movement scale

AIT. *See* Administrator-in-training

Alzheimer's disease, 60–62, 61t, 62t

Ambulatory care, 5–6

American Association of Retired Persons (AARP), 9

American Cancer Society (ACS), 150, 150t

American Diabetes Association (ADA), 149

American Health Care Association (AHCA), 154

American Nurses' Association (ANA), 217, 221

American Nurses Credentialing Center (ANCC), 174, 175t

ANA. *See* American Nurses' Association

Analgesia
opioid, 93t, 98, 101
patient-controlled, 98, 101, 101f

ANCC. *See* American Nurses Credentialing Center

Anemia, 71

Anger, 67t

Angina. *See* Chest pain

Angiotensin converting enzyme (ACE) inhibitor, 116–17

Antibiotics, 93t, 100

Anticholinergics, 69t

Antidepressants, 59t, 93t

Antihypertensives, 93t

Antimicrobials, 110

Antipsychotics, 93t, 103

APIE note, 141

APTT. *See* Activated partial thromboplastin time

Arterial blood gases, 29

Arterial occlusion, 126–27, 127t

Arteriosclerosis, 122

Aspiration pneumonia, 76, 109

Aspirin, 89